Walid Feki
Rim Kammoun
Salma Kallel

Therapeutic education for COPD patients

Walid Feki
Rim Kammoun
Salma Kallel

Therapeutic education for COPD patients

in general medicine

ScienciaScripts

Imprint

Cover image: www.ingimage.com

This book is a translation from the original published under ISBN 978-620-6-71394-4.

Publisher:
Sciencia Scripts
is a trademark of
Dodo Books Indian Ocean Ltd. and OmniScriptum S.R.L publishing group

120 High Road, East Finchley, London, N2 9ED, United Kingdom
Str. Armeneasca 28/1, office 1, Chisinau MD-2012, Republic of Moldova, Europe
Managing Directors: Ieva Konstantinova, Victoria Ursu
info@omniscriptum.com

Printed at: see last page
ISBN: 978-620-8-39316-8

Contents

1 Introduction

Among chronic diseases, chronic obstructive pulmonary disease (COPD) is one of the main causes of morbidity and mortality in the world, with a growing social and economic burden.

It is defined as "a common, preventable and treatable disease characterised by persistent respiratory symptoms and persistent airflow limitation due to airway and/or alveolar abnormalities often caused by significant exposure to noxious particles or gases"[3].

It is a disease that has long been asymptomatic or pauci-symptomatic, and is not recognised by the general population[4] . The delay in diagnosis means a delay in overall management and is detrimental to the prognosis[5] .

Worldwide, the prevalence of COPD has been rising steadily for the past 30 years, with more than 64 million patients and more than 3.2 million deaths in 2015, i.e. 6% of the adult population and 9 to 10% of the over-40s[6] Tunisia is no exception to this general trend, with a COPD prevalence of 7.8%[7] .

COPD patients, like all chronic patients, often find it very difficult to adhere fully to their treatments and to the advice of their carers [1,3].

Hence the role of Therapeutic Patient Education (TPE), which is aimed at patients with a chronic disease for whom learning health skills and behaviours is essential. Its aim is to make patients more autonomous by making it easier for them to adhere to prescribed treatments, thereby improving their quality of life[9].

TVE is currently the subject of various research projects. Its definition and application are evolving. Similarly, the guidelines for the management of chronic diseases give an essential place to TVE in the management of the disease. In France, for example, therapeutic education is cited even before pharmacological treatments in the management of type 2 diabetes, according to the French High Authority for Health (HAS) in its guide "Affection Longue Durée 8"[10].

The benefits of TVE for COPD patients are less clear-cut[11,12], but are sufficient to justify its application, particularly as part of a respiratory rehabilitation programme[13]. This will enable patients to delay the complications inherent in their disease and reduce their dependence by enabling them to integrate their disability into their daily lives.

Although TVE has begun to be practised regularly in specialised hospital departments in North African countries [14], it seems important that this discipline should be practised by general practitioners (GPs), who are the coordinators of the care pathway and the most frequently consulted by COPD patients [15,16].

To our knowledge, the practice of ETP among Tunisian COPD patients by GPs has not been evaluated. Hence the idea of carrying out a survey of GPs in the liberal sector of Sfax in order to meet the following objectives:

1- Evaluating GPs' views on TVE in COPD
2- To evaluate the practice of TVE by GPs with COPD patients.
3- To assess GPs' theoretical knowledge and level of involvement in the management of COPD patients.

The results will be used to develop new ways of improving the management of COPD patients and the integration of therapeutic education.

2 SUBJECTS AND METHODS

1. TYPE OF STUDY

This is a descriptive cross-sectional study, of the CAP type. This study is conducted among a specific population to identify the knowledge (C), attitudes (A) and practices (P) of this population on a specific theme.

2. LOCATION OF THE STUDY

Our study is a survey of general practitioners in the governorate of Sfax.

3. STUDY PERIOD

The study took place over a 4-month period from 1 December 2015 to 31 Màrch 2016.

4. STUDY POPULATION

The study population consisted of general practitioners selected at random by elementary sampling from the list of general practitioners registered with the Sfax regional medical order council (CROM), and meeting the following criteria:

4.1.Inclusion criteria

- Working in the private sector
- Operating in the Sfax region
- Whatever their orientation in daily practice

4.2.Non-inclusion criteria

- Hospital doctors
- Replacement doctors

5. DATA COLLECTION

5.1.Drawing up the questionnaire

The study took the form of two questionnaires.

tS The first questionnaire is based on a survey of GPs carried out in 2011[17]. The questions are open-ended and a data collection grid has been drawn up **(Appendix 1).**

Basic epidemiological data were obtained for each doctor questioned (age, sex and medical practice characteristics). This questionnaire was used to ask GPs about :

- What is the role of the general practitioner in the management of COPD?
- Therapeutic education: Do they practise therapeutic education? If so, how? If not, why? Do they think it should be developed and how? What objectives should be achieved? Their expectations in terms of TVE in COPD.
- GPs' opinion of COPD patients: are they asking for TVE? Why do they want it?

A total of 8 to 10 questions were asked during the interview.

Í3 The Bristol COPD Knowledge Questionnaire (BCKQ)[18] is the second questionnaire devoted to the knowledge of general practitioners, translated into French and accompanied by a grid of correct answers. **(Appendix 2).**

It comprises 65 items with a simplified 3-item response ("true", "false", "don't know").

The first 2 items concern general knowledge about COPD: some epidemiological data, screening and diagnostic methods, etc.

- Three items focusing on knowledge of different clinical signs
- Five items assessing their skills in relation to therapeutic modalities,
- Two items relating to primary and secondary prevention (focusing on smoking cessation and vaccination)
- An item on respiratory rehabilitation emphasising the role of physical activity in COPD.

5.2.Contact with doctors

5.2.1. The first stage

The doctors were contacted by a telephone call informing them that they would be carrying out a survey on a topical medical subject as part of a medical thesis. The doctors were then asked to let us know by telephone whether they agreed or refused to take part.

5.2.2. The second stage

The doctors who gave us their agreement were called to choose a suitable time to receive the questionnaire, answer it and hand it in to the investigating doctor within a period specified by the respondent (maximum one week). The time was chosen according to the most suitable period of availability for the doctor, i.e. outside a consultation.

6. STATISTICAL STUDY

- Data from the complete forms were entered and analysed using SPSS II version 20.0 software.
- Incompletely completed forms were discarded.
- Numerical values were expressed as mean plus or minus standard deviation.
- The association between categorical variables was calculated using Fisher's corrected Chi2 test for small numbers.
- Comparisons between quantitative variables were made using Student's T-test.
- Significance is acquired for a $p < 0.05$ for all statistical tests.

3 RESULTS

1. ANALYSIS OF PARTICIPATION

1.1.Participation rate

Of the 100 doctors initially contacted, 85 agreed to take part in the survey. Eighty completed the questionnaire correctly, giving an overall participation rate of 80%. The five incomplete forms were discarded.

1.2.Non-respondents

Doctors who did not reply to the questionnaire were divided into two categories: Those who declined to take part in the study when first approached. There were 15 of them. The reasons given were as follows:

- Too many demands and lack of time (for 3 doctors)
- Refusal to respond to medical theses (for 1 doctor)
- Lack of interest in the subject of COPD (for 1 doctor)
- Secret barrage (for 3 doctors)
- Specific practice (for 2 doctors)
- Nearing retirement (for 1 doctor)
- No reason (for 4 doctors)

There were 5 doctors who did not complete the questionnaire forms correctly, and whose forms were subsequently discarded. **(Figure 1)**

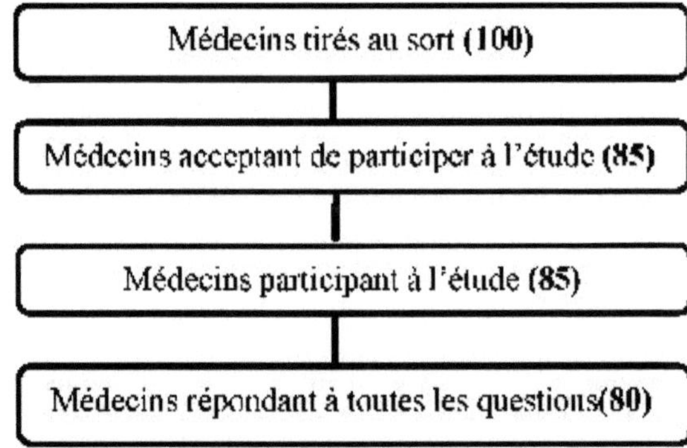

Figure 1: Distribution of doctors by participation rate

2. PROFILE OF DOCTORS WHO ANSWERED CORRECTLY

2.1.Age and gender of doctors

2.1.1. Age :

The average age of the doctors included in the study was 49, with extremes ranging from 30 to 65. The two most common age groups were [36-45] and [46-55] **(Figure 2).**

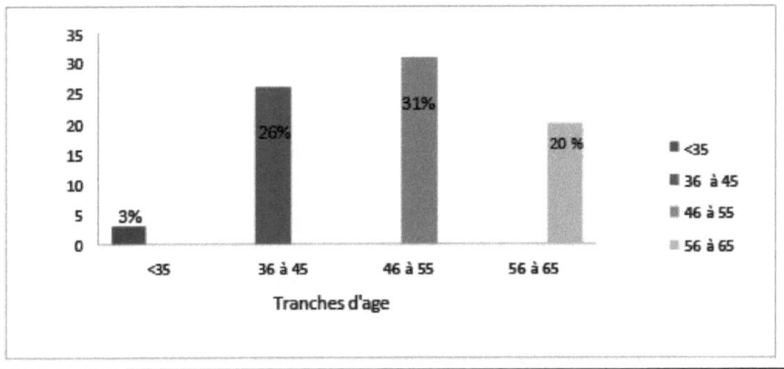

Figure 2:Breakdown of doctors by age group

2.1.2. Type

The majority of doctors surveyed were men (71%), with an estimated sex ratio of 2.4 (**Figure 3**).

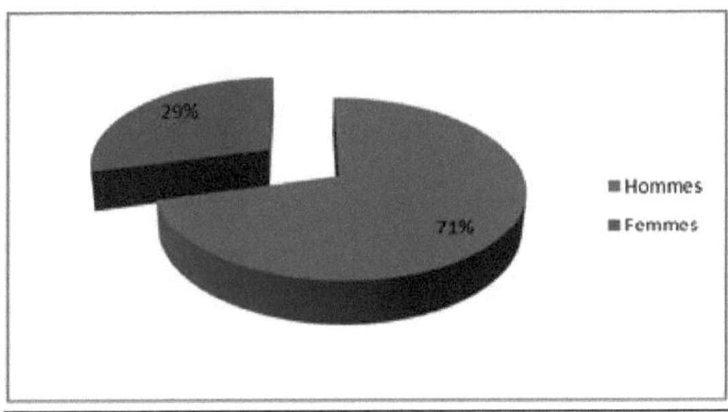

Figure 3:Breakdown of doctors by gender

2.3.Professional characteristics of doctors

2.3.1. Place of work

97% of GPs practised in urban areas.
(**Figure 4**).

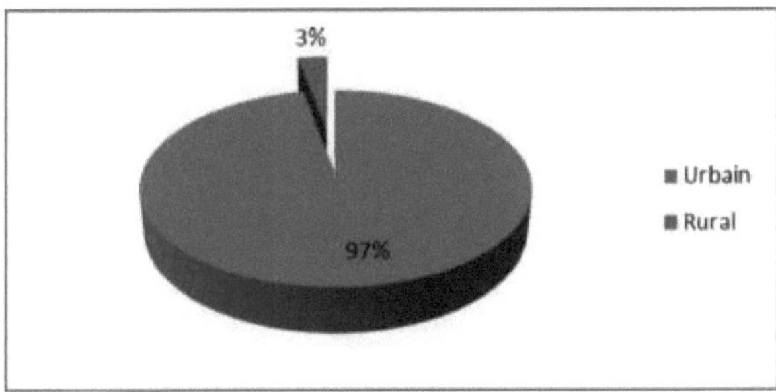

Figure 4:Breakdown of the series by place of practice

2.3.2. Type of practice

Most of the doctors surveyed practise in private practices (**Figure 5**).

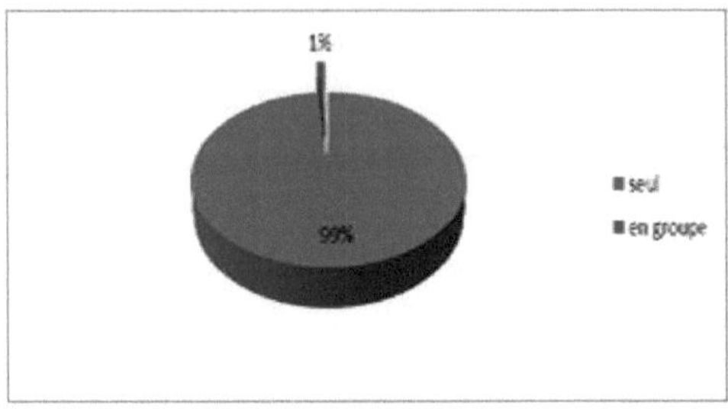

Figure 5: Breakdown of the series by type of practice

2.3.3. Specialist diplomas for general practitioners

In order to clarify the specific areas in which GPs work, they were asked a question about the postgraduate qualifications they had obtained. Homeopathy and aesthetic medicine were the most common. **[Table I]**

Table I: Specific practices of the doctors surveyed

Specialised diploma	Workforce
Aesthetic medicine	4
Homeopathy	3
Geriatrics	2
Phytotherapy	2
Diet	2

3. THEORETICAL KNOWLEDGE OF BPCO

Doctors were asked a number of questions relating to COPD, assessing several areas.

The rate of correct responses to the questionnaire assessing doctors' knowledge of COPD education (assessed using the BCKQ) was 72%.

3.1.General knowledge

3.1.1. Definition

When asked to characterise the term "chronic disease", 70% of GPs emphasised the notion of severity **(Figure 6).**

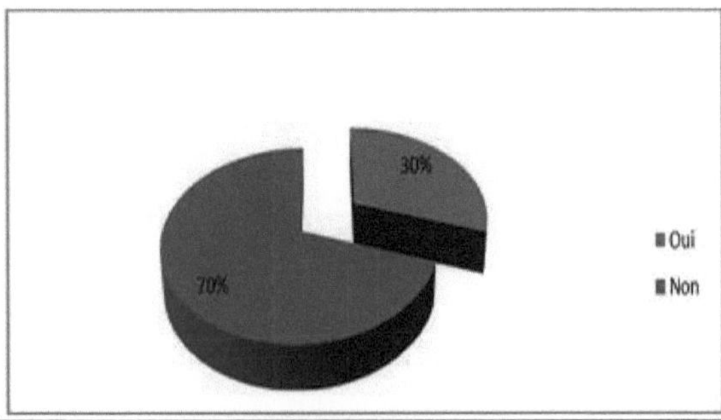

Figure 6: Doctors' answers to the question "In COPD, does 'chronic' mean severe?

means that it is severe?"

3.1.2. Risk factors

3.1.2.1. Age of onset

Sixty-one per cent of participants felt that COPD is unusual in people aged under 40, regardless of their smoking status **(Figure 7).**

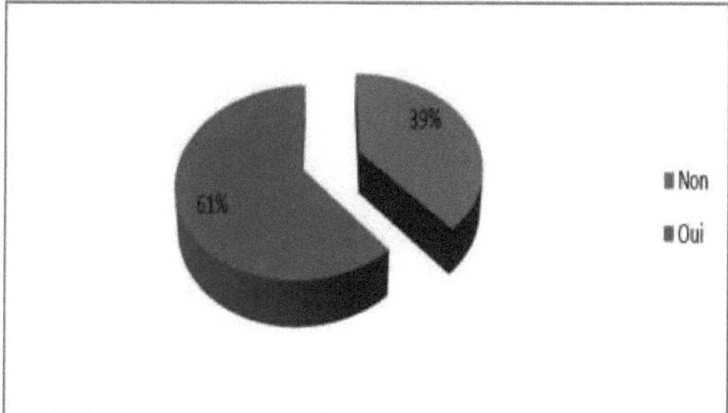

Figure 7: Distribution of doctors' answers to the question "Is COPD unusual before the age of 40?

3.1.2.2. Gender

Seventy-four of the GPs (93%) did not believe that women are less vulnerable to the effects of smoking than men. As a result, they are just as sensitive to tobacco and can develop COPD if they smoke the same amount.

3.1.2.3. Tobacco

Over 80% of COPD cases are caused by smoking, according to 91.3% of doctors.

3.1.2.4. Exhibition

COPD can also be caused by occupational exposure, according to 88.8% of the doctors surveyed.

3.1.2.5. Asthma and COPD

Long-term asthma may develop into COPD, according to 47% of respondents.

3.1.2.6. Genetic factor

To the question "Is COPD a hereditary disease? seventy-six of the participants (95%) answered no and only 4 (5%) doctors thought that COPD is indeed a hereditary disease.

3.2.Diagnosis of COPD

3.2.1. Functional and physical signs

Several functional signs were identified by the doctors surveyed. Most doctors considered cough, sputum and asthenia to be the most frequent signs accompanying a patient with COPD.

Similarly, 91% of GPs believe that wheezing is a physical sign often present in

COPD. **(Figure 8)**

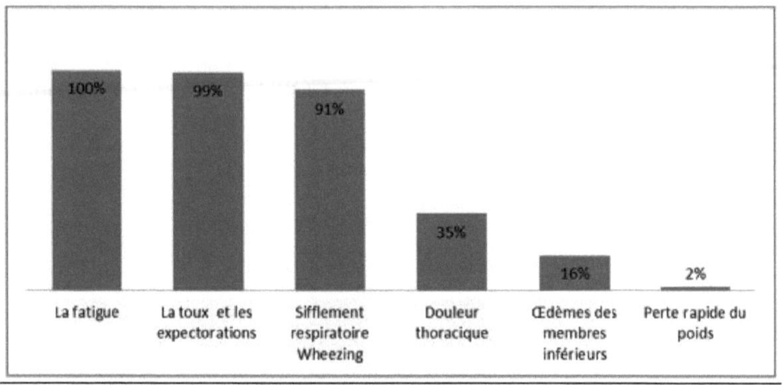

Figure 8: Distribution of functional signs according to their frequency in COPD according to GPs

3.2.1.1. Dyspnoea

- *Impact*

Several questions were asked about dyspnoea. According to 70% (n=56) of the doctors surveyed, severe dyspnoea may prevent air travel.

Seventy-nine per cent (n=63) of GPs said that dyspnoea could be made worse by eating large meals.

- *Causes*

As for the causes of dyspnoea, 67.5% of doctors said it was due to narrowing of the bronchial tubes.

Fifty-eight of the GPs (73%) considered it to be a normal response to effort. **[Table II]**

Table II: Characterisation of dyspnoea according to doctors

Questions	Yes(%)
Severe dyspnoea prevents air travel	70
Dyspnoea can be aggravated by large meals	79
Dyspnoea means that your oxygen levels are low	58
Dyspnoea is a normal response to effort	73
Dyspnoea is mainly caused by narrowing of the bronchial tubes	68
Dyspnoea reflects low oxygen levels	58

3.2.1.2. Cough

Cough is considered a frequent symptom in COPD by the majority of respondents (98%).

3.2.1.3. Sputum

Sputum is a frequent symptom in COPD, as 100% of doctors stated.

3.2.2. Additional examinations

3.2.2.1. Spirometry

To diagnose COPD, 49% of GPs used clinical criteria alone, compared with 51% who used breathing tests. **(Figure 9)**

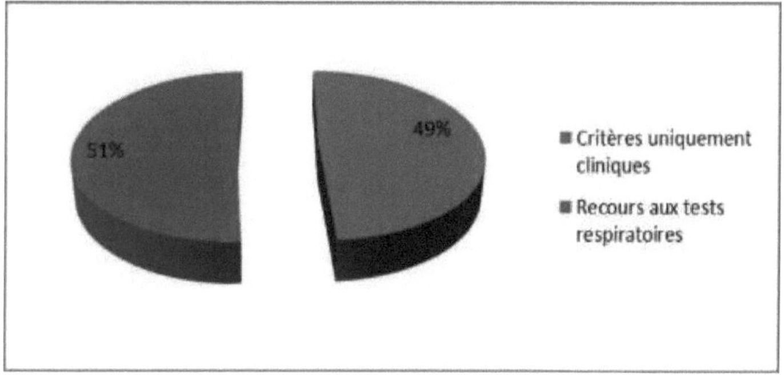

Figure 9:Distribution of responses according to the criteria adopted for the diagnosis of COPD

3.2.2.2. Pulse oximetry and blood gases

In COPD, oxygen levels in the blood are always low, according to 36% of respondents.

3.3. Treatment of COPD

3.3.1. General measures

3.3.1.1. Smoking cessation

A number of questions were asked about the benefits of giving up smoking. All our respondents are convinced that quitting smoking is always useful and that it is never too late to stop, even if the disease has already set in.

This improved COPD symptoms and slowed down other lung lesions. Lung function can recover according to 78% of our respondents **(Figure 10).**

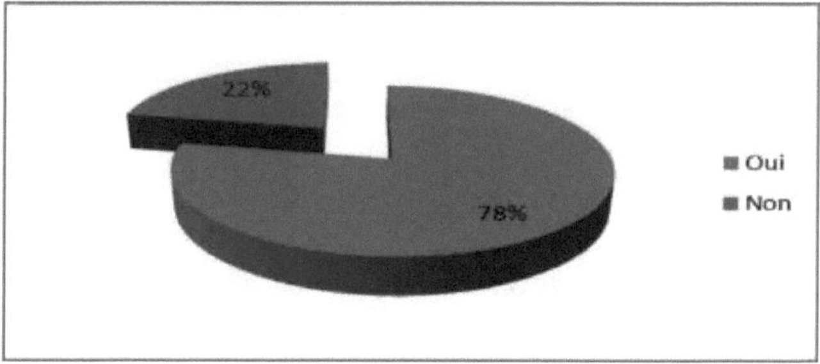

Figure 10: Does smoking cessation improve lung function?

For twenty-six doctors (32.5%), nicotine replacement therapies are only available on prescription.

3.3.1.2. Vaccination

At the same time, doctors were asked questions about vaccination. With regard to the indications for flu vaccination, all doctors considered it necessary even before the age of 65, and a booster is recommended every year according to all respondents. **[Table III]**

Table III: What is known about , the place of vaccination in COPD

Questions	Yes %
A flu booster is recommended every year	100
Influenza may develop following vaccination	66
You can be vaccinated against flu unless you are 65 or over	0
The pneumococcal vaccine protects against all forms of pneumonia	5
You can have the pneumococcal and flu vaccinations on the same day.	46

3.3.2. Medical treatment

GPs were asked a number of questions relating to the different classes of medicines used in COPD patients.

3.3.2.1. Inhaled bronchodilators

Responses varied depending on the questions asked, as shown in the table below.

following table **[Table IV]**

Table IV: Breakdown of responses from the doctors surveyed concerning bronchial tubes. inhaled dilators (BD)

Questions about inhaled BD	Yes (%)
Do all comics work quickly (within 10 minutes)?	40
Can short- and long-acting BDs be taken on the same day?	97,5
Do inhaled BD reduce sputum production?	50
Do inhalation chambers need to be dried with a towel after washing?	66
Does using an inhalation chamber increase the amount of inhaled medicine in the lungs?	85
Can trembling be a side effect of bronchodilators?	84

3.3.2.2. Antibiotic treatment in COPD

Responses concerning antibiotic therapy were distributed as follows: **[Table V]**

Table V: Breakdown of responses from doctors surveyed concerning antibiotics

Questions	Yes (%)
To be effective, the course of antibiotics should last at least 10 days?	62.5
Can overuse of antibiotics lead to resistant bacteria?	100

Do antibiotics eradicate all lung infections?	0
Is antibiotic treatment necessary for all exacerbations, even mild ones?	35
Should you seek advice if taking antibiotics is associated with severe diarrhoea?	53,8

3.3.2.3. Corticosteroids

TS **Corticoi'des orals**

- Indications and contraindications

According to 11% of respondents, the use of oral corticosteroids strengthens the muscles.

The coexistence of pulmonary superinfection is considered an absolute contraindication to the prescription of oral corticoids by 46% of doctors.

To the question "Is there an indication for oral corticosteroids whenever there is an exacerbation?", 43.8% of our respondents answered yes.

- Secondary effects

All GPs believe that the risk of long-term side-effects from corticosteroids is lower with short courses of treatment than with continuous (long-term) treatment.

Among these side effects, malabsorption is a frequent side effect of corticosteroid use according to 37.5% of doctors.

Forty-one GPs (51%) felt that oral corticosteroids can contribute to an increase in appetite.

3.3.2.3.2. Inhaled corticoids

Differing opinions on the use of inhaled corticosteroids were reported by the doctors surveyed. All the data are given in the following table: **[Table VI].**

Table VI: Breakdown of responses concerning inhaled corticoids

Questions	Yes (%)
Inhaled corticoids can be taken even if you have prescribed oral corticoids.	87,5
Inhaled corticoids can relieve dyspnoea rapidly	46 ,2
The inhalation chamber reduces the risk of contracting oral	49
thrush	29
Inhaled corticoids should be taken before bronchodilators	65
Inhaled corticosteroids improve lung function in COPD	

1.4.Exacerbations

1.4.1. Relationship between exacerbation and infection

COPD exacerbations are not always of infectious origin, according to 84%

(n=67) of doctors.

When doctors were asked about the signs suggestive of a pulmonary infection, the responses were summarised in the following table: **[Table VII].**

Table VII: Signs associated with bronchial superinfection

Questions	Yes (%)
Lung infections often cause haemoptysis With lung	18
infections the sputum is usually coloured (yellow or green)	become 97
Lung infections are always associated with fever	
3	

1.4.2. Management of sputum

To reduce sputum production, doctors suggested respiratory physiotherapy in 81% of cases and bronchodilators in 50% of cases. **(Figure 11)**

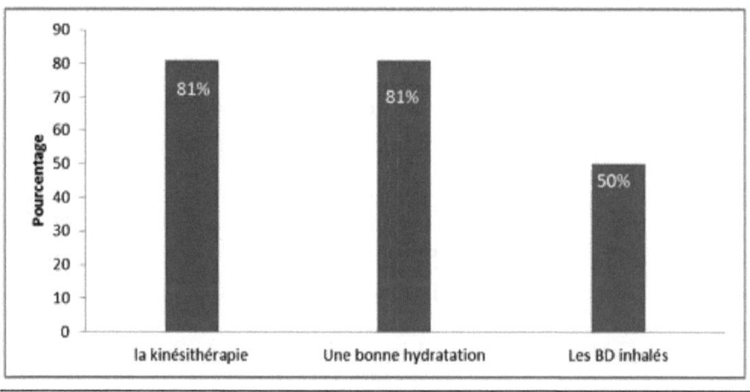

Figure 11: Distribution of responses concerning therapeutic methods used to reduce sputum production.

1.5.COPD and physical activity

1.5.1. Benefits and harms of physical rehabilitation

The majority of doctors surveyed believe that physical activity in COPD patients is beneficial. According to 82.5% (n=66), it helps maintain bone density, and 91.3% (n=73) believe that it relieves depression. On the other hand, 21.25% (n=17) of the doctors considered that sporting activity was harmful to the lungs of COPD patients and should therefore be avoided. **[Table VIII]**

Table VIII: COPD and physical activity :

GPs' views on physical activity	Yes(%)
Exercise should be avoided as it is harmful to the lungs	21
Exercise can help maintain your bone density	83
Exercise helps relieve depression	91

Exercise should be stopped if it makes the patient dyspnoeic69

1.5.2. Type of exercise

According to 86% (n=67) of participants, walking contributes better to physical rehabilitation after exercise than other respiratory exercises.

4. THERAPEUTIC EDUCATION OF GENERAL PRACTITIONERS FOR PATIENTS WITH BPCO

4.1.The role of the general practitioner in the management of patients with COPD?

According to 86% of GPs surveyed, the GP's role is to monitor and treat the disease. This is followed by screening, prevention (79%) and management of acute episodes (77%). **(Figure 12).**

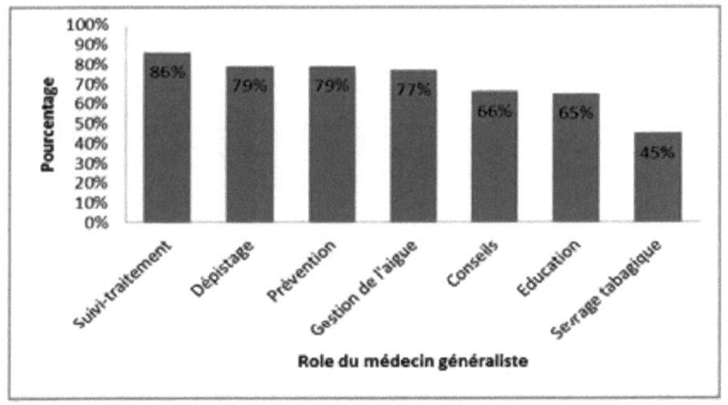

Figure 12:Breakdown of responses concerning the role of GPs in COPD management

4.2.Therapeutic education

4.2.1. In theory

According to the doctors surveyed, GPs and lung specialists should be the primary players in TVE (96% and 87% respectively). **(Figure 13).**

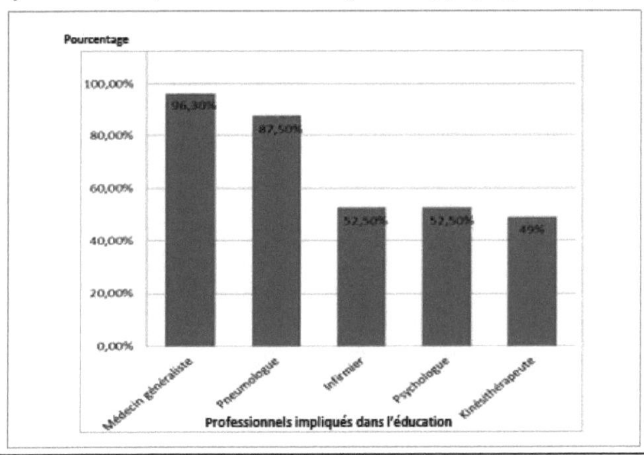

Figure 13: Ranking of professionals who should provide TVE, according to the GPs questioned.

4.2.2. In practice

Fifty-four GPs (67%) provided therapeutic education to their COPD patients. **(Figure 14)**

According to 52% of GPs, they are the key players in COPD. According to 23% of respondents, referral to a lung specialist is essential for diagnosis. Management in collaboration with the respirologist was cited by 46% of respondents.

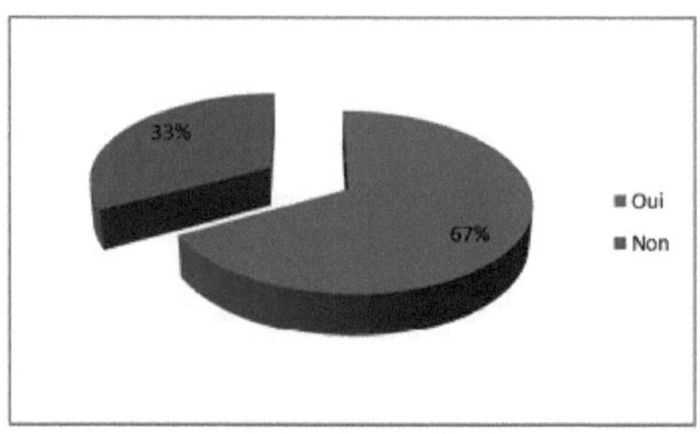

Figure 14: Percentage of GPs providing TVE to COPD patients

4.2.3. Therapeutic education methods

4.2.3.1. Place of therapeutic education practice

Therapeutic education is practised by 94% of doctors in their practices. **[Table IX]**

Table IX: Location of education provided by general practitioners

Location	Percentage
Cabinet	94
Hospital	2
Surgery and hospital	4

4.2.3.2. Other proposed venues

Other places have been mentioned by some doctors as possible sites for education **[Table X]**.

Table X: Other places for therapeutic education mentioned by GPs

Other proposed venue for TVE	Percentage (%)
Dedicated centre	27,5
Media	5
Training seminars	2,5
Home	2.5

4.2.3.3. *Structures offering therapeutic education*

For the group of doctors practising TVE, they were asked about the existence of a specialised structure offering TVE, and their answers were compiled in the following table:

[Table XI]

Table XI: Responses to the question "Is there a structure offering TVE in Tunisia?

Structures offering TVE	Workforce	Percentage (%)
No	47	58.8
COPD asthma school	2	4.1
Ariana Withdrawal Centre	1	1.3
Charles Nicolle Smoking Cessation Centre	1	1.3
Pneumology Department Sfax	2	2.5

4.2.3.4. *Patient support*

According to 62% of doctors, education took place when the patient was accompanied. **[Table XII]**

Table XII: Accompanying the patient during the education process

Is the patient accompanied?	Percentage (%)
No	19
Yes	62
The 2 possibilities	19
Total	100

4.2.3.5. Regularity of education

Education is most effective when carried out on a regular basis. This was the opinion of 85% of doctors who practised it. **[Table XIII]**

Table XIII: FTE rhythm

Pace of education	Percentage (%)
Irregular	15
Regular	85
Total	100

4.2.3.6. *Frequency of education*

Education usually takes place when patients attend their regular appointments. For our doctors, patients consult every 3 months, at which time education is carried out in 83% of cases. 15% of doctors took advantage of the exacerbation to further educate their patients. **[Table XIV]**

Table XIV:Frequency of therapeutic education for COPD patients

Frequency of education	Percentage (%)
During exacerbations	15

3 months		83
6 months		2
Total	100	

4.2.4. Aims of therapeutic education

According to the doctors surveyed, the main aims of therapeutic education are to stabilise the disease (46.3%) and avoid exacerbations (46.2%). **(Figure 15)**

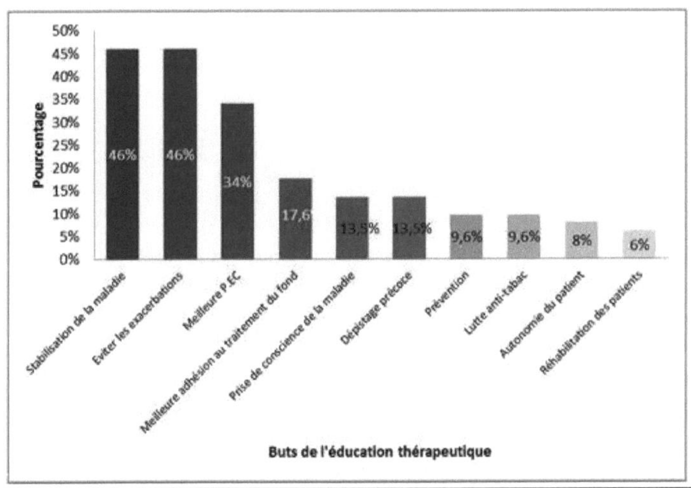

Figure 15: Goals of therapeutic education according to the doctors surveyed

4.2.5. Therapeutic education tools

According to the doctors surveyed, the therapeutic education tools needed are essentially the follow-up booklet and visual aids. **[Table XV]**

TableXV: Suggested TVE tools

Therapeutic education tools	Percentage (%)
Follow-up booklet	66
Visual support	60
Evaluation questionnaire	48

4.3.GPs' expectations of therapeutic education

To the question "What do you expect from therapeutic education? The responses were summarised in the following table **[Table XVI]**.

Table XVI: Expectations of GPs in the EPT

GPs' expectations of ETP	Percentage (%)
Primary prevention, better care to reduce overall healthcare costs	46
Raising patients' awareness of the ETP process	21,3
Raising awareness of the disease (Raising awareness via the media and organising public awareness days)	7,5

4.4.The role of COPD patients in the education process

4.4.3. Do GPs think patients want TVE treatment?

According to the doctors questioned, and based on their experience, 56% (n=45) of doctors believe that patients prefer a management approach that includes therapeutic education **(Figure 16).**

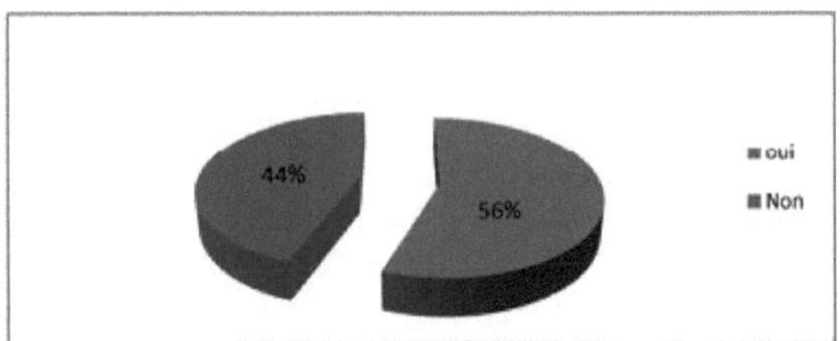

Figure 16: Do patients ask for TVE, according to general practitioners

4.4.4. The objectives of therapeutic education to be acquired by the patient

Regarding the priority objectives to be acquired by the patient, the majority of respondents cited awareness of the disease (97.5%) and knowledge about the disease (75%). **[Table XVII]**

TableXVII: Objectives of therapeutic education to be acquired by the patient

Objectives	Percentage (%)
Awareness of the disease	97,5
Knowledge about the disease	75
Improve their disease management skills	62,5

4.4.5. Benefits of therapeutic education for patients

Patients' expectations of ETP are summarised in the following table **[table XVIII].**

TableXVIII: Benefits of therapeutic education for patients

Expectations	Percentage (%)
Symptom relief	53,5
Management of acute exacerbations	43,8
Prevention	41.3
Self-management	18,8

4.4.6. Reasons for patients' lack of demand for ETP

Sixty-four percent of doctors explained that, in their opinion, patients do not seek therapeutic education because they are not aware of their illness, which is consistent with the priority objective to be achieved (Table XVII) of "raising awareness". The idea of difficult management, linked to a particular patient profile, also emerges (11% of doctors questioned). **[Table XIX]**

Table XIX: Reasons found for patients' lack of demand for ETP

Patient reasons by GP	Percentage(%)
Lack of awareness and therapeutic education	64
Stubborn patient refusing to stop smoking	11
Neglect of the disease	11
Denial and refusal to explore	8
Lack of culture and low socio-economic level	6
Total	100

5. DOCTORS NOT PRACTISINGEDUCATION THERAPEUTIC

Thirty-three percent of our respondents did not practise therapeutic education. They were asked other questions.

5.2.Should it be done?

All the doctors who did not practise therapeutic education thought that it should be done. To promote it, doctors stressed the need for continuing education for GPs (40%), the creation of dedicated centres (21.3%), the creation of weaning centres (11.3%), remuneration for GPs (2.5%) and insurance for COPD and this type of therapeutic education by the national health insurance funds (2.5%).

5.3.Why don't you practise therapeutic education?

Doctors gave two reasons for not practising TVE: those relating to patients and those relating to the doctors themselves. These different reasons are listed in the table below. **[Table XX]**

Table XX: Reasons for doctors not practising TVE

Causes	Percentage (%)
Lack of awareness and cooperation	27
Lack of time	19
Consultation unless exacerbation	19
Few patients	15
Patient refusing to stop smoking	15,5
Lack of training and no dedicated centre	15,5
Specialist case	7,7
Patient adheres to treatment without worry	7,7
Pessimism about any TVE programme	3

1. ANALYSIS OF PARTICIPATION

1.1.Participation rate

The percentage of participation in our study was 80%. This percentage is similar to that reported in other studies: 76% in the study by J.Foucaud et Coll[19], carried out among GPs in the Bordeaux urban community, but higher than the participation of doctors in the Godenir study carried out in the Chambéry basin in France, with a rate evaluated at 35% [17]. This shows the interest shown by our GPs in the various health surveys.

1.2.Non-respondents

In some studies, too many requests and lack of time were the main reasons preventing the doctor from cooperating with the investigator[17]. **[Table XXI]**

Table XXI: Reasons for non-respondents

Reasons for not responding	Godenir [17]	Our study
Lack of time	34	20
No reason given	11	26
Secretariat dam	5	20
Specific exercise preventing practice of general medicine	14	13
Few COPD patients	5	6
Early retirement	-	6
Refusal to answer thesis questionnaires	-	6
No respondent after 3 contact attempts	27	-

2. PROFILE OF DOCTORS WHO HAVE ADEQUATELY

2.1.Age and gender of doctors

2.1.1. Age

The age and length of time that doctors have been in practice are characteristics that are always sought in surveys of doctors. A doctor's age may reflect his or her experience.

Thus, Elmjendel et al, in their study evaluating the quality of COPD management by GPs in central Tunisia, reported a length of practice ranging from 11 to 20 years[15] with an age range varying from 35 to 54 years, a characteristic not sought in our study.

The average age of the 80 doctors in our study was 49, with extremes of 30 and 65. This average age is also close to that reported by J.Foucaud et Coll [19] 45.5 years, Godenir [17] 48.2 years, Raynaud 51 years [20].

2.2.Professional characteristics of doctors

2.2.1. Place of work

With regard to the distribution by environment (urban or rural), comparison is made difficult by the lack of existing data available. That said, only 3% of doctors in our study practise in rural areas, so they are very probably under-represented. This is due to a selection bias linked to the centralisation sites and probably to the urbanisation rate of the Sfax region, estimated at 62% according to the latest demographic indicators published in 2015 by the National Institute of Public Health[21].

Table XXII]

Table XXII: Physicians' place of practice

Physicians' place of practice	Urban % of total	Rural
GODENIR study [17]	53,30	46,70
Our study	97	3

2.2.3. Specialist qualifications of general practitioners

GPs are seeking to acquire additional qualifications in spite of being general practitioners. ***[Table XXIII]***

Table XXIII: Specialist qualifications of doctors

Diplomas	Foucaud[19] % %.	Our % study
Aesthetic medicine	-	3,2
Homeopathy	-	2,4
Geriatrics	-	1,6
Nutrition	3	1,6
Phytotherapy	-	1,6
Sports medicine	11	-
Mesotherapy	3	-

3. OBSTRUCTIVE CHRONIC LUNG DISEASE

3.1.Epidemiology

3.1.1. Prevalence

Existing data on the prevalence of COPD vary considerably due to differences in survey methods, diagnostic criteria and analytical approaches[22-24]. [**Table XXIV**]

Table XXIV:Prevalence of COPD

Study	Country	Year	Prevalence(%)
WHO[6]	World	2004	9 - 10
Platino[25]	Latin America	2004	7,8 - 19,7
Roche et al [26]	France	2012-2013	7,5
Landis et al [27]	Europe, Asia, USA	2012-2013	7-9
Daldoul et al [7]	Tunisia	2015	7,80

3.1.2. Mortality

From 6th place in 1990, COPD is now the 4th leading cause of death worldwide according to the WHO. It is expected to become the third leading cause of death in 2030[28] . This justifies the choice of our study.

Almost 90% of COPD deaths occur in low- and middle-income countries [28]. **[Table XXV]**

Table XXV: COPD mortality rates

Study	Year	Country	Mortality (%)
WHO [28]	2015	North America	3,70
		Europe China	3,40 4,00
Hajem INSP [29]	2013	Tunisia	1,50

3.2.Doctors' knowledge of COPD

3.2.1. Definition

The definition of COPD has changed in recent years. Recently, the Global Obesity and Lung Disease (GOLD) report from a panel of international experts defined COPD as "a common, preventable and treatable disease characterised by persistent respiratory symptoms and persistent airflow limitation due to airway and/or alveolar abnormalities often caused by significant exposure to noxious particles or gases"[3].

So COPD is not synonymous with emphysema or chronic bronchitis.

For our doctors, the question about the definition was not explicit, since our questionnaire only looked at doctors' opinions about the term "chronic disease". We found that the word chronic meant severe according to 70% of GPs.

3.3.Risk factors for COPD

3.3.1. Factors assessed by the Bristol Questionnaire (BCKQ)

3.3.1.1. The role of lung ageing

According to various studies, age has been identified as a causal factor in COPD[30- 32].

In the Latin American project (PLATINO)[25], the prevalence of COPD increased sharply with age, with the highest prevalence in people over 60.

3.3.1.2. Influence of gender

Most long-standing studies have reported that the prevalence and mortality of COPD are higher in men[25]. In our country, men suffered more often from COPD than women (86% vs. 13%, respectively)[7,31].

Based on recent European data, the prevalence of COPD is becoming almost equal in men and women, probably reflecting changes in smoking patterns [27]. Among the countries where gender is not associated with COPD prevalence are Austria [32] and Italy [33].

Other studies have suggested that women are more sensitive to the effects of tobacco smoke than men, leading to more severe disease for an equivalent amount of cigarettes consumed [34-37].

In our study, 92% of respondents felt that women and men were equally vulnerable to the effects of smoking.

3.3.1.3. Smoking

Throughout the world, smoking is considered to be the most common risk factor for COPD. In fact, COPD is linked to smoking in 80 to 90% of cases [38] .

Cigarette smokers have a higher prevalence of respiratory symptoms, impaired lung function and a higher mortality rate than smokers of other types of tobacco[39,40].

In China, Yin P. et al have shown that passive exposure to cigarette smoke can also contribute to respiratory symptoms and COPD [41].

3.3.1.4. Genetic factors

Genetic risk factors are increasingly well documented. The role of alpha-1 anti-trypsin (AAT), a major circulating inhibitor of serine proteases, is now well established [42].

Single genes, such as matrix metalloproteinase 12 (MMP12), have also been linked to reduced lung function [43].

However, it remains unclear whether these genes are directly responsible for COPD or are merely markers of causal genes[44,45].

3.3.1.5. Occupational exposure

Several studies have incriminated the role of occupational exposure in the genesis of COPD. Some of these studies are summarised in the following table:**[Table XXVI].**

Table XXVI: Role of occupational exposure in the development of COPD

Studies	Years	Fraction of COPD attributable to work exposure (%)
Hnizdo et al [46]	2002	19,2
American Thoracic	2003	10-20

Studies	Society [47]	
Gan et al [48]	2013	6-15
Paulin et al [49]	2015	38

In our study, 88.8% of the doctors incriminated the role of occupational exposure to dust in the development of COPD.

3.3.2. Factors not assessed by the BCKQ

3.3.2.1. Atmospheric pollution

It is a recurring question whether air pollution is a factor in the aggravation or development of COPD.

A project carried out in eight European cities in 2001 studying the short-term effects of particles on health showed that for a 10 gg/m3 increase in exposure to solid ultrafine particles and nanoparticles (PM10), there was a 1% increase in the risk of hospitalisation for COPD in subjects aged over 65. Significant relative risks with the other pollutants NO2, O3 and SO2 have also been found[50,51].

3.3.2.2. Socio-economic status

Low socio-economic status is associated with an increased risk of developing COPD [52,53], although it is not clear whether this is related to overcrowding, poor nutrition, infections or other socio-economic factors.

3.3.2.3. Lung development

This factor may be related to birth weight [54,55].

3.3.2.4. The role of infections

- **Respiratory infections in childhood**

In the European Respiratory Health Survey carried out between 1991 and 1993 on 4636 subjects, it was shown that a history of severe respiratory infection in childhood is associated with impaired lung function in adulthood[33]. In terms of COPD, susceptibility to infection plays a role in exacerbations, but not in the development of the disease.

- **HIV infections**

In America, HIV infection has been shown to accelerate the onset of smoking-related emphysema and COPD [56].

- **Tuberculosis**

In Australia, tuberculosis has also been identified as a risk factor for COPD[57].

3.4.Diagnosis

COPD is suspected when there is evidence of exposure to a risk factor, and functional and physical signs. The diagnosis is confirmed by spirometry [23].

3.4.1. Functional signs

The most common respiratory symptoms are dyspnoea, cough and/or sputum.

These symptoms may be under-reported by patients[3].

3.4.1.1. Dyspnoea

sSTerminology and assessment

It is the main symptom of COPD. Dyspnoea is a major cause of the disability and anxiety associated with the disease [58], beginning with progressive breathlessness on exertion and then at rest. Dyspnoea is assessed using a number of scales. The most widely used is the mMRC scale.

£3 *Aetiologies*

The mechanisms of dyspnoea are varied:

***J* Static and/or dynamic pulmonary hyperinflation**

The reduction in airway calibre following inflammation progressively traps air during exhalation, leading to hyperinflation. Static hyperinflation reduces inspiratory capacity and is generally associated with dynamic hyperinflation during exercise[59,60].

***J* Peripheral muscle dysfunction**

COPD reduces active mobility and leads to skeletal muscle dysfunction[61]. It is characterised by muscle atrophy, a reduction in muscle strength and a drop in oxidative capacity, leading to exercise intolerance and deconditioning in patients, which further exacerbates dyspnoea[62].

***J* Central mechanism**

This is an imbalance between increased ventilatory demand and insufficient or ineffective ventilatory response[63].

In our study, questions were asked about the causes of dyspnoea via BCKQ and the link between dyspnoea and normal exercise response in COPD patients?"

3.4.1.2. Chronic cough and sputum

Ö **Chronic cough** is often the first symptom of COPD and is frequently regarded by the patient as an expected consequence of smoking and/or environmental exposures. Chronic cough in COPD is often productive [64].

Sputum

Patients producing large volumes of sputum may have underlying bronchiectasis. The presence of purulent sputum reflects an increase in inflammatory mediators[65]. A change in sputum colour may suggest a bacterial infection, although the association is relatively weak [66,67].

In our study, cough and sputum were considered the most frequent symptoms by all the doctors surveyed.

To reduce sputum production, doctors suggest physiotherapy in 81% of cases and bronchodilators in 50% of cases.

+ **Other symptoms.**

- Fatigue, weight loss and anorexia are common problems in patients with severe and very severe COPD[68,69]. They have prognostic significance and may also be a sign of other diseases, such as tuberculosis or lung cancer, and should therefore always be investigated [70,71]. For all our doctors, fatigue was a common symptom, but only 2% of doctors felt that weight loss was present.

• Coughing spells can also cause rib fractures, which are sometimes asymptomatic. In our study, 35% of respondents felt that chest pain is a common symptom in COPD.

3.4.2. Physical examination

The physical examination may be normal at the beginning or show bronchial rales [72,73]. At a later stage, other signs may be noted, reflecting the progressive nature of the disease.

Wheezing is an intermittent symptom that can vary from day to day and even within the same day. It takes the form of wheezing that can be heard without a stethoscope.

In our study, 91% of GPs saw wheezing as a sign often present in COPD.

3.4.3. Additional examinations

3.4.3.1. Spirometry

The GOLD criteria show that spirometry is of crucial importance in the diagnosis of COPD[3]. It represents the most reproducible and objective measure of bronchial obstruction [74,76].

The spirometric criterion for limiting airflow remains a fixed post-bronchodilator ratio of FEV1/FVC <0.70 = Tiffneau ratio.

However, it should be noted that the use of the fixed FEV1/FVC ratio to define airflow limitation may result in a more frequent diagnosis of COPD in the elderly, and a less frequent diagnosis in adults <45 years of age.

GOLD therefore recommends the use of the lower limit of normal (LON) for FEV1/CVF, particularly in patients aged under 30 and over 50[77].

Although spirometry is required for a diagnosis of COPD, 49% of our doctors made a positive diagnosis of COPD without recourse to these respiratory tests and were satisfied with the semiological criteria.

This finding raises the question of the difficulty for GPs to diagnose COPD in routine practice, as has been mentioned in other studies [17,19,20].

3.4.3.2. Imaging

ü Chest X-ray

A chest X-ray is not useful for establishing a diagnosis of COPD, but it is useful for ruling out differential diagnoses of chronic dyspnoea (pulmonary fibrosis, bronchiectasis, abnormal heart shape).

In patients with COPD, chest X-rays may show signs of thoracic distension or areas of hyperclarity indicative of emphysema ö **Chest CT scan**

Although not systematically recommended, thoracic CT scans are useful for

- detection of bronchiectasis
- suspected underlying neoplasia.
- Observe the emphysema lesions and their distribution for the purposes of decide on surgery (lung reduction, resection of bullae, lung transplantation) [78,79].

3.4.3.3. Oximetry and arterial gas

This measurement can be used to assess a patient's arterial oxygen saturation and the need for additional oxygen therapy. Pulse oximetry should be used to assess all patients with clinical signs suggestive of respiratory failure or right heart failure. If peripheral arterial oxygen saturation is less than 92% arterial or capillary, blood gases should be assessed [80,81].

In our study, a misconception adopted by 36% of doctors was in favour of the presence of constant hypoxaemia regardless of the stage of the disease.

3.4.3.4. Alpha-1 anti-trypsin assay

Alpha-1 antitrypsin deficiency can be detected in young patients (< 45 years) with a predominantly emphysematous phenotype and/or a family history of non-smoking COPD [82].

3.4.3.5. 6-minute walk test

This test is indicated for assessing the degree of exercise tolerance.

3.4.4. Assessment and classification of COPD

COPD is currently classified into 4 stages A, B, C and D. This classification is based on three parameters: risk of exacerbation, CAT and the Mmrc scale: **(Figure17).**

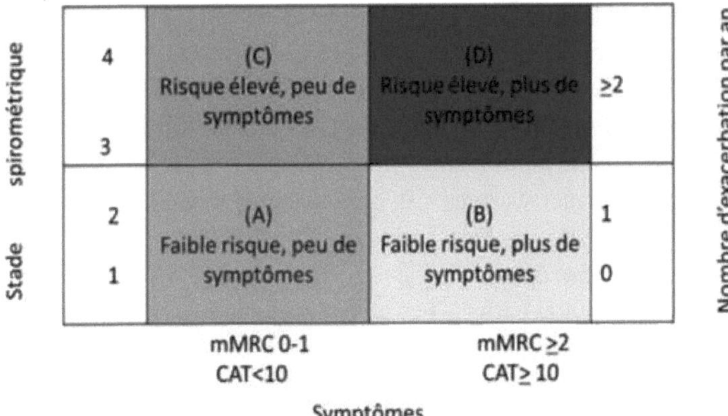

Figure 17: Combined assessment of COPD severity [3].

3.5.Impact

3.5.1. Assessment of quality of life in COPD patients

3.5.1.1. Aims of the assessment

The aim is to assess the physical, mental and social aspects of an individual's state of health[83]. Assessing quality of life is also of interest to the healthcare authorities, especially as it is better correlated with the use of healthcare facilities (hospitalisation rates, emergency room visits, frequency of exacerbations, etc.) than the usual physiological parameters [84-87].

3.5.1.2. Valuation methods

Quality of life assessment is based on general or COPD-specific questionnaires measuring the physical, psychological and social factors associated with the disease [88]. The best known of these are the St George's (SGRQ) [89], the SF36[90] and the CAT[91].

3.5.2. Factors influencing patients' quality of life

Some studies[92,93] report that the quality of life of COPD patients is impaired by a number of factors[94].

3.5.2.1. Poor compliance with treatment

Using the SF36 and SGRQ, Spencer et al [93] demonstrated that quality of life deteriorated more rapidly in patients in the placebo group compared with the fluticasone group.

3.5.2.2. Frequency of exacerbations

People with stable COPD always have significantly higher quality of life scores than those suffering from an exacerbation[95].

3.5.2.3. Smoking

Smoking has been associated with poorer quality of life in COPD populations. According to Spencer et al[93], when patients who smoked were assessed, their SF-36 scores were lower than those of non-smokers.

3.5.3. Comorbidities

COPD is considered to be a systemic disease, with extra-pulmonary manifestations contributing to morbidity and mortality [96]. These include :

3.5.3.1. Metabolic pathologies

COPD significantly increases the risk of developing diabetes, heart disease and stroke[97,98].

3.5.3.2. Undernutrition

Undernutrition in COPD patients has a poor prognosis. It is detrimental to both respiratory and non-respiratory muscle function [69].

3.5.3.3. Osteoporosis

Osteoporosis is directly related to systemic inflammation in COPD[99], in particular IL6 and TNF alpha, which are also key cytokines in COPD[100].

Osteoporosis is a source of vertebral fractures in patients with moderate to severe COPD.

3.5.3.4. Anemia

Although COPD is quite rightly a chronic respiratory pathology which predisposes to polycythemia, several studies have recently come to support the presence of anaemia in a significant number of these patients[101].

It is associated with an increase in the rate of hospitalisations, a reduction in exercise capacity and is a predictive factor for mortality [102].

3.5.3.6. Psychopathological comorbidities

It is estimated that the prevalence of depression varied from 6 to 80% in COPD patients, with an average of around 40% in the majority of the most comprehensive studies [103].

Anxiety and depressive symptoms increase the frequency of exacerbations [104] and hospitalisations, and prolong the length of hospital stays [105,106].

3.5.3.7. Peripheral neuropathy

Recently, peripheral neuropathy has been incriminated as being responsible for an impact on exercise capacity and quality of life in patients with moderate to very severe COPD [107].

3.5.4. Respiratory effects

In the study by Voll-Aanerud et al, the link between respiratory symptoms and reduced quality of life was observed [108].

3.5.5. Cardiac repercussions

COPD patients are at high risk of cardiovascular disease[109,110]. These are among the main causes of death in this population[111].

The cardiovascular diseases most frequently associated with COPD are pulmonary arterial hypertension, heart failure, atherosclerotic coronary disease, stroke, cardiac arrhythmias and dilated cardiomyopathy[112,113].

3.6.Therapeutic strategies

These strategies are largely based on the GOLD recommendations[3].

3.6.3. COPDstable

3.6.1.1. General measures

3.6.1.1.1. Smoking cessation

Smoking cessation is the main therapeutic measure capable of influencing the natural history of the disease. Smoking cessation is beneficial for all COPD patients, whatever their age or stage of the disease.

In our study, the opinions of our doctors were all favourable. Quitting smoking is always useful. According to all our GPs, it improves COPD symptoms, slows down other lung damage and reduces the risk of co-morbidities such as cardiovascular disease.

According to the Fletcher curve (**Appendix 3**), stopping smoking allows a physiological decline to be restored (10 to 20 ml/year) without recovering the lost function. It also illustrates that it is never too late to stop smoking, even if there are already significant signs of COPD[114].

For example, 78% of our doctors thought that it would be possible to recover respiratory function after stopping smoking.

3.6.1.1.2. Vaccination

J Flu vaccine

Despite the almost unanimous recommendation that COPD patients should receive an annual influenza vaccination, very few randomised controlled trials have evaluated the effects of vaccination in these patients.

In our study, the GPs were well aware that this vaccine is recommended every year, but a significant proportion (66%) thought that influenza could develop following this vaccination, which is not theoretically the case.

J Pneumococcal vaccine

Pneumococcal polysaccharide vaccine is recommended for all patients aged 65 or over, and for younger COPD patients with significant concomitant medical conditions, including chronic heart or lung disease[115].

In our study, 95% of GPs felt that the pneumococcal vaccine does not protect against all types of pneumonia.

This has been demonstrated by certain large-scale studies [116].

3.6.1.2. Drug treatment

Background pharmacological treatment of COPD is used to reduce the symptoms, frequency and severity of exacerbations and improve exercise tolerance [118].

3.6.1.2.1. Bronchodilators

Two families of BD can be used: anticholinergics and beta-2-agonists.

ΐϊ **Beta-2-agonists (LABA)** are effective on :

- the symptoms of the disease, mainly dyspnoea.
- exercise capacity
- reducing the number of exacerbations
- improving quality of life.

Long-acting anticholinergic drugs

Long-acting antimuscarinics (LAMAs) block the bronchoconstrictive effects of acetylcholine on M3 muscarinic receptors expressed in the smooth muscles of the airways[118,119]. LAMA-based treatments (tiotropium) improve patients' symptoms(120) and reduce exacerbations and hospitalisations [121].

Combination of bronchodilators

Anticholinergics and beta-2-agonists have equivalent overall efficacy in COPD. They also have an additive bronchodilator effect without increasing any side-effects[122].

Many LABA /LAMA combinations are available as fixed combinations.

A study in patients with a history of exacerbations showed that a LABA/LAMA combination was more effective than LABA alone or in combination with inhaled corticosteroids CI/LABA in preventing exacerbations[123,124].

3.6.1.2.2. Inhaled corticoids

In vivo data suggest that the dose-response relationships and long-term safety (>3 years) of inhaled corticosteroids (ICS) in COPD patients are unclear and require further investigation[125].

Most studies have shown that regular treatment with ICS alone does not alter the long-term decline in FEV1 or mortality in patients with COPD[126]. 65% of GPs believed that ICS improves lung function in COPD. This also reflects their lack of knowledge of the therapeutic effects of these molecules.

Long-term use of IC may lead to certain side effects, in particular pneumonia, oral candidiasis, hoarseness and percutaneous echymosis[126].

The fixed combination of beclometasone, formoterol and glycopyrronium has confirmed its efficacy in the management of severe to very severe COPD. Patients have fewer exacerbations than with tiotropium and FEV1 improves[127,128].

3.6.1.2.3. Oral glucocorticoids

Oral corticosteroids have no role in the background treatment of COPD due to a lack of benefit and a high rate of long-term systemic complications.

3.6.1.2.4. Methylxanthines

The exact effects of xanthine derivatives remain controversial[129,130].

Theophylline improves inspiratory muscle function [129] and produces greater improvements in FEV1 and breathlessness than salmeterol alone [131,132].

3.6.1.2.5. Phosphodiesterase-4 (PDE4) inhibitors

The main action of PDE4 inhibitors is to reduce inflammation [133]. Thus, roflumilast reduces exacerbations in patients with

Severe to very severe COPD[134]. Effects on respiratory function are also observed when roflumilast is added to LABA[135].

3.6.1.3. Respiratory rehabilitation

The term "respiratory rehabilitation" refers to a comprehensive, multidisciplinary approach to COPD. It includes :

- therapeutic patient education
- optimising pharmacological treatment
- help to stop smoking
- exercise re-training
- respiratory physiotherapy for bronchial drainage
- psychosocial care

- nutritional management

It lasts for a minimum of 6 weeks. The benefits include an improvement in exercise tolerance, a reduction in the sensation of dyspnoea, a reduction in the number and length of hospitalisations and a reduction in mood disorders such as depression and anxiety.

It is recommended regardless of the stage of the disease, as soon as there is a handicap (dyspnoea) that has not been improved by pharmacological treatment.

In our study, 21% of doctors considered that sporting activity is harmful to patients' lungs and should be avoided.

3.6.1.4. Instrumental treatment

3.6.1.4.1. Oxygen therapy

It is indicated in situations where it has been shown to be effective in terms of survival.

- PaO2 < 55 mmHg measured in room air, at a distance from an exacerbation,
- PaO2 <60 mmHg with presence of :
  - signs of pulmonary hypertension
  - polycythemia
  - signs of right heart failure

3.6.1.4.2. Non-invasive ventilation

Non-invasive ventilation in the stable state is indicated in certain situations.

According to Murphy et al, in their study of patients with persistent hypercapnia following an acute exacerbation of COPD, the addition of non-invasive home ventilation delayed readmission within 12 months[136].

3.6.1.5. Indications for referral to a lung specialist

Patients must be referred to a respirologist.

- At the time of diagnosis
- If respiratory failure worsens, to reassess management
- In case of diagnostic doubt
- To discuss the indication for oxygen therapy or non-invasive ventilation
- To assess the possibility of volume reduction surgery or transplantation (patients <65 years old).

According to our doctors, 23% of them believe that recourse to lung specialists is justified. Management in collaboration with the pulmonologist was cited by 46% of respondents.

3.6.2. Exacerbation of COPD

3.6.2.1. Drug treatment

3.6.2.1.1. Short-acting beta-2 agonists (SABA)

It is the essential treatment for all exacerbations [137,138].

Inhaled administration should be preferred, as it is more effective than the systemic route, with fewer side effects. The use of an inhalation chamber or nebuliser is recommended.

According to 85% of respondents, the inhalation chamber increases the amount of medication inhaled and can prevent oral thrush (49%).

3.6.2.1.2. Antibiotics

The use of antibiotics in exacerbations remains controversial, but is justified in the event of an exacerbation. Treatment should be assessed after no more than 3 days and prescribed for an average of 7 days.

In our study, doctors felt that to be effective, a course of TBA should last at least 10 days.

3.6.2.1.3. Oral corticoids

Oral corticosteroids reduce recovery time and hospital stay by approximately 24 hours, and improve FEV1 and arterial hypoxaemia [139].

Forty-four per cent of GPs believe that OCs are indicated for every exacerbation.

3.6.2.2. Instrumental treatment

3.6.2.2.1. Controlled oxygen therapy

Its objective is to achieve saturation levels of between 88% and 92%.

3.6.2.2.2. Non-invasive ventilation

It is indicated in hospitals in cases of :

-respiratory acidosis (pH<7.35 and/or PaCO2>6.0 kPA, 45 mmHg)

-and/or severe dyspnoea associated with signs of respiratory muscle fatigue.

4. THERAPEUTIC EDUCATION

4.1.World Health Organisation (WHO) definition

In 1998, the WHO proposed a definition of TVE, which is still relevant today: "Therapeutic patient education is a continuous process, integrated into care and centred on the patient. It comprises organised awareness-raising, information, learning and psychosocial support activities concerning the disease, the prescribed treatment, care, hospitalisation, other conceived care institutions, and the patient's health and illness behaviours. It aims to help patients and their families to understand their illness and treatment, cooperate with their carers, live as healthily as possible and maintain or improve their quality of life. Education should enable patients to acquire and maintain the resources they need to manage their lives with the disease in the best possible way".

4.2.Stages of therapeutic education

According to the WHO recommendations of June 2007, TVE should be carried out in 4 stages [140].

4.2.1. Balance sheet

This involves talking to the patient to determine their level of awareness of their condition, as well as their needs and expectations of the ETP programme.

4.2.2. Contract

Ask the question: what does the patient still have to learn?

Based on the objectives defined, formulate the skills to be acquired.

4.2.3. Learning

Educational activities can be carried out in groups or individually. A theme is developed during each session. (Knowledge of the mechanisms of the disease, smoking cessation, treatments, the benefits of physical activity, etc.).

4.2.4. Assessment

Evaluation is an essential component of therapeutic education. It focuses on the patient's expectations, quality of life and knowledge acquired. It is carried out at the beginning and end of each session, to determine the focus of the sessions and the progress made.

4.3.The role of the general practitioner in the management of COPD

4.3.1. Monitoring and treatment

With regard to the tasks that GPs can carry out, the majority of respondents (86%) felt that GPs can monitor and treat the disease, while slightly fewer (65%) thought that they could carry out educational consultations. Monitoring this chronic disease is ranked as the second most important role after screening in the study by

Godenir [17]. According to Foucaud [19], GPs see their role as one of prescribing rather than educating.

4.3.2. Acute management

This dynamic approach to care, which is widely practised in general practice (77% of GPs did so), is also favoured by an increased, even unique, demand from patients to treat the acute phases of their illness.

4.3.3. Prevention

The prevention of complications in COPD is part of TVE [17,140].

According to our study, 79% of GPs consider prevention to be one of their concerns. A similar result was found in various studies.

4.3.4. Screening

4.3.4.1. State of the place

COPD is a chronic disease, with little or no symptoms for a long time. Patients do not seek help specifically for respiratory complaints because their symptoms are long-standing, trivialised and neglected. The delay in diagnosis leads to a delay in overall management and adversely affects the patient's prognosis, leading to chronic respiratory failure. Roche et al. have shown that there is a marked under-diagnosis of the disease, suggested by the high proportion of subjects with a chronic cough and/or dyspnoea who have no diagnosed respiratory disease[5], which places the general practitioner in the front line for detecting COPD, particularly in relation to risk factors[141].

4.3.4.2. Screening for COPD by general practitioners

For our doctors, 79% thought that screening for COPD was one of the GPs' roles. However, almost half of GPs saw no need to use breathing tests.

Screening for the disease therefore seems insufficient. The use of some breath-measuring equipment requires only brief training, which could be incorporated into continuing medical education (CME)[142]. in order to encourage GPs to equip themselves with a spirometer and produce good quality "flow/volume" curves in the surgery.

This can be achieved by organising "prevention consultations" for people aged over 40 with risk factors (smoking and/or occupational exposure) or by setting up a programme, as was the case in France, where a programme of actions has already been implemented in favour of COPD (2005-2010), entitled "Understanding, preventing and better managing COPD"[13].

4.3.5. A dynamic ({'education in the background in COPD

In our study, GPs ranked education as the 6th most important task, cited by 65% of them. We note a similarity with the results of the study by Foucaud et al [19], where the analysis of the discourse revealed a dynamic more focused on prescribing than on advice and education. Similarly, in the Godenir study, education was ranked 4th among GPs' missions.

4.4.Therapeutic education for COPD patients

4.4.1. Professionals to involve

The recommendations of the WHO working group on therapeutic patient education suggest that education should be provided by trained healthcare professionals: general practitioners, specialists, nurses, physiotherapists, pharmacists, psychologists and social workers [143].

In our study, 96% of the doctors questioned thought that GPs could play a central role in TVE. This high level of confidence in the GP's role is very encouraging for the development and integration of TVE into primary care.

Specialists come second (87%), with no practitioner believing that they play no role at all. Next in order of importance are nurses (53%), followed by psychologists (53%) and physiotherapists (49%).

4.4.2. GP practices

Less than two thirds of doctors (67%) said that they themselves provide therapeutic education, which is a rather low figure given the 96% of doctors who believe that GPs can play a central role in TVE. It is therefore interesting to consider the obstacles to implementing TVE in general practice.

Our results are far different from those of the GODENIR study, where the percentage of doctors practising ETP was no more than 3%[17].

4.4.3. Methods of ¡'education

4.4.3.1. Where ¡therapeutic education is practised

According to the doctors, 94% of them provide TVE in their surgeries. This choice of place by our doctors, probably due to a lack of regional care structures, is nevertheless included in the recommendations for rehabilitation offered in consultation, during hospitalisation, according to Chambouleyron et al [9].

The dedicated centre, although it does not exist in this regional sector, is cited as a possible place for TVE by 28% of GPs. This supports the need to structure TVE. In his study, Reynaud describes referring patients to dedicated centres as the most appropriate solution [20].

However, in the Foucaud et al study, the most suitable places according to independent GPs were the practice and the hospital, with a clear preference for the hospital, leading to the conclusion that this was also an implicit educational approach [19].

It therefore seems essential to set up a coordinated network to promote patient education, with reciprocal cooperation and exchanges between community doctors and hospitals.

4.4.3.2. Supporting patients during the education process

In our study, the patient was accompanied in 64% of cases. This support is an excellent opportunity to ensure that the patient's family and friends are involved in the TVE process.

According to Foucaud et al, the concern of family and friends was well noted in their study [19] and suggests that management should include family and friends.

4.4.3.3. FTE frequency

According to the example of the ETP programme applied at the Chambéry hospital centre in France, illustrated by Godenir in her study [17], any approach to educating patients requires a timetable for educational sessions. The first session is organised while making contact with the patient, with a flexible timetable in a climate of empathy and trust, in order to establish an educational diagnosis with the patient. Three to four sessions are then organised, lasting an hour on average, and ideally repeated every fortnight.

In our study, we note that our doctors' practices are occasional, since TVE is only practised at the time of consultations with a frequency of less than or equal to once a quarter (83

The practice is either very common (15% of GPs use it only when consulting a patient for an exacerbation) or very occasional (15% of GPs use it only when consulting a patient for an exacerbation).

4.4.4. Aims of therapeutic education

According to the WHO, the aim of TVE is to enable patients to acquire two types of skills: Self-care skills: to modify the effect of the disease on their health.

4- Coping skills: skills that enable people to control and direct their lives and acquire the ability to live in and change their environment [20].

In our study, the main aims of TVE in the doctors' responses were to get patients to adhere to their disease-modifying treatment (according to 17% of GPs) and to prevent exacerbations as far as possible (46%).

On the other hand, the role attributed to TVE in the promotion of early screening, prevention, or even tobacco control remains modest with consecutive proportions (13.5%, 9.6%, 9.6%).

4.4.5. Therapeutic education tools

According to Godenir(17) , certain tools are used in educational sessions:

J **The "image folder"**: illustrating pathophysiology, aggravating factors, how treatments work, breathing and relaxation techniques, etc.

J **The logbook** is rarely used, because in practice patients find it difficult to keep track of their symptoms, exacerbations and the progress of their disease. The hypothesis is that the daily reminder of the disease generates a certain amount of anxiety.

■*S* Interactive CD-ROMs

***J* Information booklets**

In our study, these tools are essentially represented by the follow-up booklet and the visual aid for more than 60% of our GPs. Next came the evaluation questionnaire, which 48% of GPs felt was necessary.

The use of the Fletcher curve is also a good tool for illustrating the progression of the disease and the benefits of smoking cessation, but none of our GPs mentioned it [114].

4.4.6. Effectiveness of TVE in COPD

The gain brought by TVE in terms of COPD was an avenue of research in various studies. Lenferink et al in their search [144] conducted in the Cochrane Specialist Register in May 2016 (22 included studies involving 3,854 participants with COPD with variable follow-up from two to 24 months). Studies comparing the effectiveness of an action plan for acute exacerbation with usual care, were able to consider these action plans as a key component of COPD self-management interventions.

However, McGeoch et al in their prospective study [145] conducted in general practice over 12 months in 2006, comparing usual care with usual care combined with structured education on the use of a written self-management plan and patient-initiated courses on antibiotics and oral corticosteroids, found that knowledge of self-management was higher in the intervention group but had no effect on quality of life, health utilisation, mental health or patient satisfaction.

4.4.7. Impact of therapeutic education on overall health costs

Rasekaba et al [146] in their comparative study between 2 groups of patients (one with TVE for 1 to 2 months and a group without TVE or a duration of no more than 0 to 3 weeks of education) were able to conclude that the total cost associated with the use of hospital care fell from 130,000 dollars to 7,500 dollars for the group with TVE with a rise from 77,700 dollars to 101,200 dollars for the 2nd group without TVE.

4.4.8. How to improve TVE

4.4.8.1. Improving training

This is indeed an essential condition for leading and designing a TPE programme, as described in the HAS recommendations. A non-exhaustive list of skills is needed by healthcare professionals to implement therapeutic patient education in a multidisciplinary way: interpersonal skills, teaching and leadership skills, methodological and organisational skills, biomedical and care skills.

Indeed, a significant improvement in GPs' knowledge, with correction of all critical errors and improved attitudes towards teaching and implementation in clinical practice, has been noted in various studies [147].

4.4.8.2. Organising continuing training

The WHO recommends two types of in-service training:

- Short courses of 50 h to 100 h delivered by training organisations and universities (university diplomas);
- long courses at master's or doctorate level.

For healthcare professionals who are already trained (doctors, pharmacists, nurses, chiropodists, dieticians, physiotherapists, etc.), the need is to acquire new educational skills, which can be acquired through short courses (a few days), university diplomas or longer courses such as bachelor's or master's degrees.

4.4.8.3. The creation of dedicated centres

A structured TVE programme represents a reference framework for implementing a personalised programme for each patient. It defines, in a given context, who does what, for whom, where, when, how and why TVE should be carried out and evaluated. The WHO also recommends[140]:

- WHO Member States "to reorganise and restructure healthcare systems to implement the therapeutic patient education approach".

- healthcare manufacturers "to sponsor healthcare centres involved in research into therapeutic patient education".

4.4.8.4. Raising patients' awareness so that they adhere to ETP programmes

In COPD, the onset of the disease is insidious. Awareness of the disease is difficult, complicating the application of TVE (148) (149). In order to provide education, the patient must be :

- aware that it has a problem
- convinced that we can solve this problem
- convinced that he can solve the problem himself (this is the notion of "internal locus of control" described in psychology)

4.4.8.5. Raising awareness of the harmful effects of smoking, including the creation of smoking cessation centres

No TVE would be complete without addressing the harmful exposure caused by smoking.

4.4.8.6. GP remuneration

This could be another way of motivating doctors to practice TVE. In Switzerland, for example, there is no specific remuneration for doctors who decide to carry out educational activities. On the other hand, the Swiss system remunerates the practitioner according to the length of the consultation, in 5-minute increments, which allows the necessary time to be devoted to education[17].

4.4.8.7. Ensuring that TVE is covered by national health insurance funds or even learned societies

The WHO recommends [140]:

- insurance companies "to include therapeutic patient education as a reimbursable expense for insured patients".

4.5.The role of the COPD patient in the education process

4.5.1. Do GPs think that patients want TVE?

Patients need TVE, but not all of them seek it. According to the results of our questionnaire, 60% of the doctors questioned believe that patients have only a very limited knowledge of their illness, but that this does not mean that they are seeking information. Forty-five per cent of doctors deplored this. This result corroborates certain findings in the literature, such as those of Godenir et al[17,150]. In the latter qualitative study of GPs, 70% of patients did not request TVE. This view of patients appears to be incorrect, and it would be interesting to know the proportion of GPs who inform their COPD patients of the existence of specialised education, and to ascertain from patients the actual number of refusals.

4.5.2. The objectives of therapeutic education to be acquired by patients, according to doctors

Awareness and knowledge of the disease were cited as priority objectives for patients by the majority of respondents (98% and 75% respectively).

A study of the general population carried out between 2002 and 2012 concluded that only 8.6% to 17% were aware of the existence of COPD [4,151]. A French study carried out in 2004 showed that 8% of respondents, out of a sample of 2758, knew the term "COPD" but 93% knew the term chronic bronchitis and 69% knew the term emphysema [5,152].

This lack of knowledge makes awareness of the disease a key objective of TVE.

Developing skills in disease self-management was also seen as an objective for more than half the doctors questioned (62.5%).

4.5.3. Patients' expectations of ETP

According to Bellamy and Smith [141], moderate to severe COPD patients are the ones who request information on physical exercise and symptoms of the disease. In our study, 55% of patients requested TVE.

According to our GPs, the main concern of COPD patients is symptom relief (54%), which is in line with Foucault's study [19]. A smaller proportion (18%) thought that these patients were asking to acquire self-management skills. Thus the "planned and organised transfer of skills from the carer to the patient-health partner" which usually characterises TVE did not appear in our study. This finding confirms that educational management is not yet really integrated into therapeutic management [153].

4.5.4. Reasons for patients' lack of demand for ETP

4.5.4.1. Lack of awareness

One of the striking points is that a significant proportion of patients seem not to have understood the chronic nature of their disease, with a real ignorance of the evolution and complications of COPD (60% of doctors replied that patients do not request therapeutic education because they are not aware of their disease). This motivates doctors to rank awareness of the disease as the primary objective of TVE (cited by 98% of doctors).

4.5.4.2. Patients are highly addicted to tobacco

According to the majority of GPs, COPD patients generally refuse to stop smoking, sometimes denying their illness and refusing to be explored, which corroborates the results of the literature [17,20].

4.6.Doctors not practising TVE

4.6.1. Barriers to the practice of TVE

4.6.1.1. Patient-related difficulties

If we analyse the reasons for GPs not practising TVE, we find that patient-related reasons top the list:

4.6.1.1.1. The patient's "lack of awareness" of his or her condition and its difficulties

This is the main reason cited by doctors (27%), which is indeed a primary objective of TVE. This is akin to denial, an unconscious and long-lasting process whereby people refuse to accept the reality of chronic illness. This has been found in other studies, such as that by Gibbons et al.

[154] and that of Halpern [155]. Similarly, Barbara P and Peter C in their study in which the participants (doctors and nurses providing primary care for chronic diseases including COPD) report that their intervention in the management of COPD is always confronted by patients' inability to report symptoms of COPD [156].

4.6.1.1.2. Patient refusing to stop smoking

This refusal on the part of patients to stop smoking is a cause which undermines any effort at TVE and will make it very difficult for patients to become involved in a therapeutic education approach. Our doctors explain this by the notion of difficulty (for 15.5% of them) which is associated with the idea of a "patient profile", often "passive", which seems to be linked to smoking. Walters N and Coleman T report that patients do not believe very much in the benefits of stopping smoking [157].

The role of the treating physician is crucial at this level, to help patients accept their illness and identify a problem by supporting them in their search for a solution.

4.6.1.2. Lack of time

According to 19% of respondents, their only obstacle to practising TVE was lack of time, which was mentioned as the second most important reason. This was presented in various studies as the main reason [17,19]. This problem is often found in general practice. The average consultation time for GPs in France is 17 minutes [158]. This time also varies considerably from one doctor to another, and even from one patient to another, but remains between 15 and 30 minutes in most consultations. Furthermore, patients with one or more chronic pathologies often represent a large proportion of a patient base: it is impossible to carry out a TVE for all of them, but this is not insurmountable in view of the expected benefits of this practice, which may in time make it possible to save time.

4.6.1.3. Consultation unless exacerbation

Because of the unconscious and long-lasting process of denying the reality of chronic illness, 15.5% of doctors reported that patients only consult a doctor in the event of an exacerbation.

4.6.1.4. Few COPD patients in the patient population

The fact of having few people with COPD in their patient base is a less frequently cited reason (15% of GPs) but, here again, does not justify exempting them from one of the resources in the therapeutic arsenal, namely TVE.

4.6.1.5. Lack of training

The lack of training is much less frank than the lack of time or the lack of patient adherence: while 16% of doctors do not give enough importance to TVE due to "lack of training", 40% of them insist on the need for continuing education for GPs in terms of COPD and TVE, which corroborates with Reynaud's study [20] where the doctors questioned also mentioned their lack of training in TVE. In fact, the time devoted to TVE courses was reduced to just a few hours during their studies [159].

4.6.1.6. Lack of a network and ¡no dedicated centre for TVE issues

There is a form of education that can be described as informal, and which is distinct from therapeutic patient education. This practice may continue, but it does not justify exempting patients from a more structured form of education that has proved its worth, particularly in terms of benefits for quality of life.

Yet this is a justification put forward by 15% of GPs. What's more, educational activities are poorly valued in the current healthcare system. According to HAS recommendations in France in June 2007, TVE must be structured and well organised if a real education programme is to be established[140].

4.6.1.7. More questionable reasons

According to 7.7% of our doctors, TVE is seen as the specialist's business. For them, it is a field monopolised by lung specialists. 7.7% of doctors report that they do not practise TVE because patients certainly adhere to their treatment on their own.

Pessimism about any TVE programme" was expressed by a
the only doctor interviewed.

These reasons are linked to a poor understanding of the activity and challenges of therapeutic education and a lack of information and awareness among GPs.

4.6.2. Should we do it?

Despite the significant percentage of doctors who do not practise TVE (33%), 100% of doctors are in favour of developing TVE: once again, this percentage shows the involvement of all doctors in developing TVE.

4.7.Algorithm for implementing a therapeutic education programme

With the aim of highlighting therapeutic education for COPD patients in our context, we designed this example of an approach in which the steps in blue are specific to the HAS 2007 TPE approach [140].

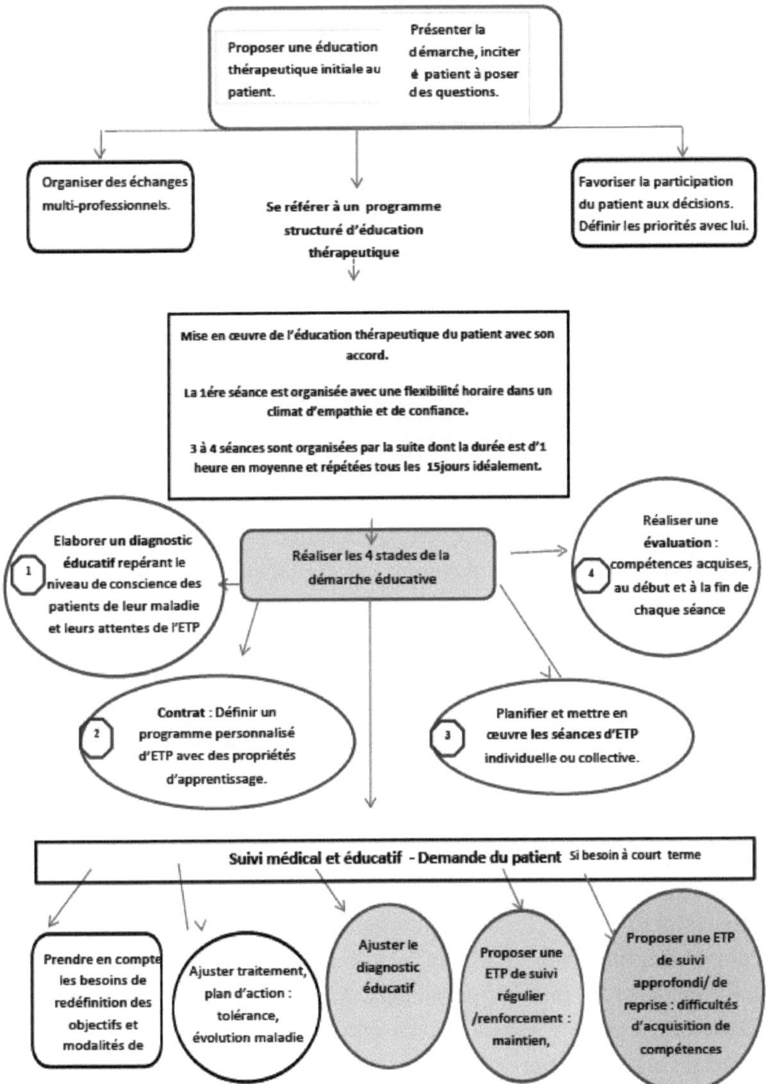

5 CONCLUSION

In the same way as drug treatment, therapeutic patient education (TPE) is now part of the "therapeutic armoury" available to doctors in the management of chronic diseases. Its aim is to improve patients' quality of life, by delegating to them some of the medical skills needed to promote a degree of autonomy and help them live better with their illness. It also responds to a public health issue linked to the growing prevalence of chronic diseases.

The incidence of chronic obstructive pulmonary disease (COPD) is rising at an alarming rate: with ¡increasing life expectancy and ¡increasing smoking rates, the risk of less regulated occupational exposure, and indoor air pollution from ¡biomass burning, COPD will be the third leading cause of death by disease by 2030. In Tunisia, the prevalence of COPD is estimated at 7.8%. COPD has a major impact on patients' quality of life, and the use of TVE is essential.

There is therefore a strong demand for COPD care in our country, a demand that is being met by a shortage of demographically-skilled care staff specialising in pulmonology.

General practitioners (GPs), who are much larger and better distributed, are the healthcare professionals most frequently consulted by COPD patients. For this reason, GPs should be the key players in the management of this disease and in the practice of TVE.

To our knowledge, the practice of TVE among Tunisian COPD patients by GPs has not been evaluated. The aim of our study was to ascertain the views of Tunisian GPs about TVE and the difficulties they experience in practising this approach, as well as to assess their knowledge and behaviour in the face of COPD.

To do this, we conducted a cross-sectional study with a descriptive CAP type in the form of a survey which took place between December 2015 and March 2016 and concerned GPs in the governorate of Sfax. Our study consisted of a survey of a representative sample of the target population, drawn at random by elementary sampling from the list of GPs that we were able to obtain from the regional council of the order of physicians. After drawing lots, we selected a list of 100 GPs. These were asked to take part in the survey; 80 (80%) of them responded favourably to our request.

For each doctor, an initial anonymous questionnaire was used to obtain basic socio-demographic data (age, sex and characteristics of medical practice), data on disease management in general practice, therapeutic education in COPD and patient demand for TVE.

The GPs' knowledge was assessed using a second scientifically validated questionnaire, the BCKQ, translated into French and comprising 65 items with a simplified 3-item response ("true", "false", "I don't know") for each question.

The average age of the GPs in our study was 49. The 46-55 age group was the most represented (31%). They were male in 71% of cases (sex ratio = 2.4). The practice area was urban for 97% of the GPs, all of whom worked in the private sector.

The rate of GPs who responded in accordance with the BCKQ's scientific data exploring knowledge about COPD was 72%.

When it comes to COPD risk factors, exposure to tobacco can cause COPD in 80% of cases, according to 91% of GPs. Indeed, worldwide, smoking is by far the main risk factor for COPD. Passive smoking is also a risk factor.

This disease is unusual before the age of 40 (61% of GPs). 93% of our doctors believe that women and men are equally vulnerable to the effects of smoking. Despite this finding being consistent with the literature, it has recently been shown that COPD can affect women in earlier and more severe forms.

Only 5% of GPs believed that COPD is a hereditary disease. Genetic risk factors are increasingly well documented, in particular alpha-1 antitrypsin deficiency, which has been clearly identified. Other genetic factors are currently being evaluated.

However, several studies in the literature have incriminated the role of occupational exposure in the genesis of COPD. In our study, 88.8% of GPs blamed occupational exposure to dust for the development of COPD.

Functional signs including cough, sputum and asthenia were considered to be common in COPD patients by most respondents. In the literature, the most common respiratory symptoms are dyspnoea, cough and/or sputum but these may be under-reported by patients.

Dyspnoea in particular is a major cause of the disability and anxiety associated with the disease, beginning with progressive breathlessness on exertion and then at rest. According to our GPs, its main mechanism is narrowing of the bronchi (68%).

To diagnose COPD, 49% of respondents relied on purely semiological criteria and 51% on breathing tests. This result, which is comparable with those of other studies, highlights the need to develop simple diagnostic methods that are easily used by GPs. According to 23% of respondents, recourse to a respirologist is essential for diagnosis.

Screening for COPD was assessed as one of the GPs' roles, but it was felt to be insufficient. Although 79% of our doctors thought that screening for COPD was one of their roles, almost half of them saw no need for breath testing. The use of some breath-measuring equipment requires only brief training and could encourage GPs to equip themselves with a spirometer and produce good-quality "flow/volume" curves in the surgery in order to screen more easily for the disease.

In terms of COPD management and general measures, our doctors were all in favour of the usefulness of stopping smoking. In fact, stopping smoking is the main therapeutic measure capable of influencing the natural history of the disease.

As far as vaccination is concerned, despite the almost unanimous recommendations that COPD patients should receive an annual flu vaccination, in our study 66% of GPs thought that influenza could develop following this vaccination, which is not theoretically true.

In terms of background treatment, 50% of GPs thought that bronchodilators were indicated to reduce sputum production.

Among the reasons for prescribing ICs, 46% of our respondents felt that ICs are indicated for the rapid relief of dyspnoea. This result is not in line with international recommendations. While most studies have shown that regular treatment with ICs alone does not alter the long-term decline in FEV1 or mortality in COPD patients, 65% of GPs believe that ICs improve lung function in COPD. This shows how little doctors know about the therapeutic effects of these drugs. What has been proven is that the combination of ICs and LABA improves respiratory function and reduces exacerbations. Overall, FEV1 improves with the fixed extrafine combination of beclometasone (CI), formoterol (LABA) and glycopyrronium (LAMA), whose efficacy has been confirmed in the management of severe to very severe COPD, with fewer exacerbations.

Oral corticosteroids have no role in the background treatment of COPD due to a lack of benefit offset by a high rate of long-term systemic complications. In our study, all doctors were aware of the long-term side-effects of OCs, although 43% felt that OCs were indicated for each exacerbation.

With regard to antibiotics, compared with the data in the literature (the average duration is 7 days), GPs felt that the minimum duration of antibiotics in the event of an exacerbation is 10 days.

COPD patients, like all chronic patients, often find it very difficult to adhere fully to their treatments and to the advice of their carers. For this reason, respiratory rehabilitation, an integral part of care, is carried out over 6 weeks for all COPD patients and includes:

- therapeutic patient education
- optimising pharmacological treatment
- help to stop smoking

- exercise re-training
- respiratory physiotherapy for bronchial drainage
- psychosocial care

In our study, we sought to assess the views of our GPs on therapeutic education in particular. They revealed an approximate vision of ETP as described in the HAS recommendations.

Analysis of the results revealed that 67% of our doctors practise therapeutic education. This rate seems high compared with other studies. But as education was ranked 6th by our GPs after monitoring and prescribing, we were able to conclude that the dynamic was more focused on prescribing than on advice and education.

With regard to the professionals to be involved in TVE, the recommendations of the WHO working group suggest that education should be carried out by healthcare professionals who are essentially trained in patient education: general practitioners and specialists, nurses, physiotherapists, pharmacists, psychologists and social workers.

In our study, the general practitioner and the respirologist ranked highest, with the GP slightly higher. Management in collaboration with the respirologist was cited by 46% of respondents. This view encourages the integration of TVE into primary care.

Various forms of education were sought. The place where therapeutic education was practised was the practice in 94% of cases. This choice of place by our doctors, probably due to a lack of regional or even national care structures, is nevertheless included in the recommendations for rehabilitation offered in consultation or during hospitalisation, according to some data in the literature. Other studies describe referring patients to dedicated centres as the most appropriate solution.

However, in order to practise TVE, a structured programme representing a reference framework for the implementation of each patient's personalised programme is recommended by the WHO. This structure is lacking in our country in terms of COPD, which is why our doctors' educational approach can be described as implicit.

With the aim of optimising and evaluating the TVE process, various tools such as image files, interactive CD-ROMs and information booklets illustrating the physiopathology, aggravating factors, mode of action of treatments, breathing and relaxation techniques are recommended in the literature. The use of the Fletcher curve is also a good tool for illustrating the progression of the disease and the benefits of smoking cessation, but none of our GPs mentioned it. In fact, more than 2/3 of respondents recommended the use of the follow-up booklet as a tool for judging the effectiveness of TVE. However, given that it is a reminder of the day-to-day aspects of the disease, it is considered to generate a certain amount of anxiety. The questionnaire for evaluating the educational approach seemed necessary according to 48% of GPs, which is in line with the recommendations.

With regard to patient demand for TVE as part of their care, the respondents thought that patients would need TVE, but not all of them sought it (45% of doctors). It appears that 60% of the doctors questioned thought that patients had only very partial knowledge of their illness. For patients seeking TVE (55%), according to the doctors, their expectations of the educational approach were restricted to symptom relief (according to 53.5% of GPs) and the management of acute exacerbations (according to 43.8% of GPs). Only 18.8% of GPs thought that their patients were seeking to acquire self-management skills.

But when asked what essential objectives should patients be aiming for? Our doctors insisted on

- Awareness of the disease (97.5%)
- Knowledge of the disease (75%)
- Their competence in terms of disease management (63%)

The objectives of doctors and patients in ETP are divergent. Thus, TVE, which is a planned and organised transfer of skills from the doctor to the patient as a health partner, is designed to reduce the gap between the doctor and the patient.

According to the WHO, the aim of TVE is to enable patients to acquire self-care and adaptation skills: skills that enable people to master and acquire the ability to live in their environment and to modify it, "to know oneself, to know how to manage one's emotions, to develop critical thinking, to set oneself goals, to evaluate oneself, to strengthen oneself". These were also the main aims of TVE mentioned in the doctors' responses, along with the need to get patients to adhere to their basic treatment (according to 17% of GPs) and to prevent exacerbations as far as possible (46%).

The role attributed to TVE by doctors in promoting early detection and prevention, and even in the fight against smoking, remains modest, with consecutive proportions (13.5%, 9.6%, 9.6%).

With regard to doctors' expectations of the education task, 46% of them expect better primary prevention and a reduction in overall health costs. The impact of TVE in reducing overall health costs has been demonstrated in the literature.

Greater patient awareness of the TVE process is also one of the expectations of 21% of respondents, and greater awareness of the disease according to 7.5% of GPs. The latter expectation is relevant in view of the lack of awareness of COPD among the general population, as shown by various data in the literature.

TVE, a process that raises awareness of the disease, will thus encourage people to consult their doctor earlier and encourage doctors to make the diagnosis at a less advanced stage.

The benefit of TVE in terms of COPD was an avenue of investigation in various studies which may have considered dedicated action plans as a key component of COPD self-management interventions. However, other studies found that knowledge of self-management was higher with TVE programmes, but had no effect on change in the respiratory questionnaire (SGRQ) assessing quality of life, health utilisation, mental health or patient satisfaction.

According to our study, all the doctors are convinced of the value of TVE and would like to see it developed in conjunction with primary care, but 33% of those surveyed did not practise TVE.

The main obstacles to this practice were difficulties in changing the behaviour of patients who were unaware of their illness (27%), time constraints (19%), the fact that patients only came for consultations in the event of an exacerbation (15.5%), the lack of training for professionals (15.5%) and the absence of a coordinated network facilitating the integration of GPs into multidisciplinary care.

There were other, more critical reasons. According to 7.7% of respondents, TVE was the specialist's business, a field monopolised by pulmonologists. Similarly, according to 7.7% of GPs, patients adhered well to their treatment and did not require TVE. One doctor expressed pessimism about any TVE programme.

These reasons are linked to a poor understanding of the activity and challenges of therapeutic education and a lack of information and awareness among GPs.

As GPs cannot implement TVE for all patients with chronic illnesses, it would seem necessary to promote collaboration with trained paramedical professionals, in private practice, or with structures created for the purpose. This will require awareness-raising and training for GPs, so that they can better understand the issues and practice of TVE, and thus better convince patients of the value of the educational approach.

Although our study provides a relevant overview of current practice, it does have certain limitations:

- This study was carried out among 80 GPs, which is a small sample. As such, it cannot claim to be representative of the population of GPs in the governorate of Sfax.
- As this is an questionnaire , there exists a bias linked toto the interviewer,

inevitable, but limited by the fact that we're talking about one and the same person.

- In addition, there is a bias linked to the geographical selection of the population, located in the governorate of Sfax.
- For the BCKQ questionnaire assessing doctors' knowledge, some therapeutic modalities are not covered.

In view of our results and the data in the literature, and despite diagnostic and therapeutic advances in the field of chronic pathologies, COPD is still a little-known pathology. And even though therapeutic education has begun to be practised regularly in specialist hospital departments in the Maghreb countries, COPD is the poor relation of TVE. Certain measures seemed important to improve the management of COPD patients by GPs, essentially the improvement of specialist medical training in terms of COPD and therapeutic education. Our analysis has shown that doctors are interested in TVE, but its role should be better defined and clearly ensured in a multidisciplinary way, including the GP, for the benefit of the patient. We therefore need to better identify the obstacles to the introduction of TVE in general practice, and to give more thought to the structural means capable of improving overall care. But we still need to set objectives that are tailored to the needs of doctors and patients?

Bibliography

1. Jaffiol C. The place of the general practitioner in the care pathway for chronic diseases in France. Int J Med Surg. 2017;4(s):14-20.
2. Jacquat D. Education thérapeutique du patient. HEGEL ISSN 2115-452X 2011 3. 2011;
3. Global Initiative For Chronic Obstructive Lung Disease 2017. http://goldcopd.org/gold-2017-global-strategy-diagnosis-management-prevention-copd/.
4. Vestbo J, Anderson W, Coxson H, Crim C, Dawber F, Edwards L, et al. ECLIPSE investigators. Evaluation of COPD Longitudinally to Identify Predictive Surrogate Endpoints (ECLIPSE). Epub 2008 Jan 23. Apr 2008;31(4):869 - 73.
5. Roche N, Perez T, Neukirch F, Carré P, Terrioux P, Pouchain D, et al. Subjects at risk of COPD in the general population: disproportion between the frequency of symptoms, their perception and knowledge of the disease. Rev Mal Respir - REV MAL RESPIR. 1 May 2009;26:521-9.
6. WHO | Chronic obstructive pulmonary disease (COPD). WHO.
7. Daldoul H, Denguezli M, Tabka Z, Harrabi I. Chronic obstructive pulmonary disease in Tunisia: prevalence and impact on daily life. Rev Mal Respir. Jan 2015;32:A84.
8. Scheen A, Giet D. Therapeutic non-compliance: causes, consequences, solutions. Rev Médicale Liège. 2010;65(5-6):239-45.
9. Chambouleyron M, Surpas P, Jacquemet S. Éducation thérapeutique des patients atteints de BPCO. Rev Mal Respir. 2005;22(5):79-82.
10. Haute Autorité de santé (HAS). Actes et prestations Affection de longue durée Diabetes type 1 et diabète de type 2.
11. Peytremann-Bridevaux I, Staeger P, Bridevaux P-O, Ghali WA, Burnand B. Effectiveness of chronic obstructive pulmonary disease-management programs: systematic review and meta-analysis. Am J Med. May 2008;121(5):433-443.e4.
12. Effing T, Monninkhof EM, van der Valk PDLPM, van der Palen J, van Herwaarden CLA, Partidge MR, et al. Self-management education for patients with chronic obstructive pulmonary disease. Cochrane Database Syst Rev. 17 Oct 2007;(4):CD002990.
13. Bertrand X. Preface by the Minister of Health and Solidarity. Rev Mal Respir. 2006;23:5-6.
14. Ben Saad H, Hamadou R, Ben Cheikh I, Chouchene A, Rejeb N, Zbidi A, et al. Respiratory rehabilitation of patients with chronic obstructive pulmonary disease: preliminary data from the Tunisian experience. J Réadapt Médicale Prat Form En Médecine Phys Réadapt. 1 Dec 2008;28(4):138-47.
15. Elmjendel I, Kacem A, Garrouche N, Gargouri I, Aissa S, Benzarti W, et al. Evaluation of the quality of management of chronic obstructive pulmonary disease (COPD) by general practitioners in central Tunisia. Rev Mal Respir. 1 Jan 2016;33(Supplement):A200.
16. Bourdillon F, Mosnier A, Godard J. Public health missions for general practitioners. Santé Publique. 2008;20(5):489.
17. Godenir B. L'education therapeutique du patient atteint de broncho-pneumopathie chronique obstructive dans le bassin chamberien: évaluation des pratiques en medecine generale et propositions pour l'avenir. 2011.
18. White R, Walker P, Roberts S, Kalisky S, White P. Bristol COPD Knowledge Questionnaire (BCKQ): testing what we teach patients about COPD. Chron Respir Dis.

2006;3(3):123-31.
19. J.Foucaud, M.Versel, O.Laugt, A.Taytard. L'éducation thérapeutique du patient atteint de BPCO:Le discours du médecin généraliste Résutats d'une analyse automatique du discours. Elseiver Masson; 2005.
20. Reynaud A. Education thérapeutique du patient BPCO en médecine générale Enquête auprès d'un groupe de médecins généralistes du Limousin. [Limousin]: UNIVERSITE DE LIMOGES Faculté de Médecine; 2014.
21. KLOUZ A, BRAYEK A, BEN AMOR N. République Tunisienne health map. 2015.
22. Mathers CD, Loncar D. Projections of Global Mortality and Burden of Disease from 2002 to 2030. PLOS Med. 28 Nov 2006;3(11):e442.
23. Halbert RJ, Natoli JL, Gano A, Badamgarav E, Buist AS, Mannino DM. Global burden of COPD: systematic review and meta-analysis. Eur Respir J. Sept 2006;28(3):523-32.
24. Quach A, Giovannelli J, Chérot-Kornobis N, Ciuchete A, Clément G, Matran R, et al. Prevalence and underdiagnosis of airway obstruction among middle-aged adults in northern France: The ELISABET study 2011-2013. Respir Med. Dec 2015;109(12):1553-61.
25. Menezes AMB, Perez-Padilla R, Jardim JRB, Muiño A, Lopez MV, Valdivia G, et al. Chronic obstructive pulmonary disease in five Latin American cities (the PLATINO study): a prevalence study. Lancet Lond Engl. 26 Nov 2005;366(9500):1875-81.
26. Roche N, Ajjouri R, Compagnon A, Van Der Molen T, Mullerova H. French data in the international Continuing to confront COPD (C2C) survey. Rev Mal Respir. 1 March 2017;34(3):180-7.
27. Landis SH, Muellerova H, Mannino DM, Menezes AM, Han MK, van der Molen T, et al. Continuing to Confront COPD International Patient Survey: methods, COPD prevalence, and disease burden in 2012-2013. Int J Chron Obstruct Pulmon Dis. 2014;9:597-611.
28. WHO | The 10 leading causes of death. WHO.
29. . Hajem S. . Specific impediments, summary of the main results for 2013 and outlook. The research and information unit on ageing and medical causes of death, national institute of public health; 2015.
30. Mercado N, Ito K, Barnes PJ. Accelerated ageing of the lung in COPD: new concepts. Thorax. May 2015;70(5):482-9.
31. Bellali H, Zaghouani R, Ben Alaya N, Chahed M. Recours aux urgences pour un motif respiratoire dans la région du grand tunis, entre 2007 et 2010. La tunisie Medicale. 2015;Vol 93 (n°07) : 465-469.
32. Schirnhofer L, Lamprecht B, Vollmer WM, Allison MJ, Studnicka M, Jensen RL, et al. COPD Prevalence in Salzburg, Austria. Chest. Jan 2007;131(1):29-36.
33. de Marco R, Accordini S, Marcon A, Cerveri I, Antó JM, Gislason T, et al. Risk Factors for Chronic Obstructive Pulmonary Disease in a European Cohort of Young Adults. Am J Respir Crit Care Med. Apr 2011;183(7):891-7.
34. Foreman MG, Zhang L, Murphy J, Hansel NN, Make B, Hokanson JE, et al. Early-Onset Chronic Obstructive Pulmonary Disease Is Associated with Female Sex, Maternal Factors, and African American Race in the COPDGene Study. Am J Respir Crit Care Med. August 15, 2011;184(4):414-20.
35. Silverman EK, Weiss ST, Drazen JM, Chapman HA, Carey V, Campbell EJ, et al. Gender- related differences in severe, early-onset chronic obstructive pulmonary disease. Am J Respir Crit Care Med. 2000;162(6):2152-2158.

36. Martinez FJ, Curtis JL, Sciurba F, Mumford J, Giardino ND, Weinmann G, et al. Sex Differences in Severe Pulmonary Emphysema. Am J Respir Crit Care Med. August 2007;176(3):243-52.
37. Tam A, Churg A, Wright JL, Zhou S, Kirby M, Coxson HO, et al. Sex Differences in Airway Remodeling in a Mouse Model of Chronic Obstructive Pulmonary Disease. Am J Respir Crit Care Med. 15 Apr 2016;193(8):825-34.
38. El Fekih L, Berraies A, Hamzaoui A, Fenniche S, Megdiche M, Boussen H. Impact du tabagisme sur les affections brochopulmonaires : Ampleur du problème. La tunisie Medicale. El Fekih;89 (n°011) : 814-819.
39. Kohansal R, Martinez-Camblor P, Agustí A, Buist AS, Mannino DM, Soriano JB. The Natural History of Chronic Airflow Obstruction Revisited: An Analysis of the Framingham Offspring Cohort. Am J Respir Crit Care Med. Jul 2009;180(1):3-10.
40. Tan WC, Lo C, Jong A, Xing L, Fitzgerald MJ, Vollmer WM, et al. Marijuana and chronic obstructive lung disease: a population-based study. CMAJ Can Med Assoc J J Assoc Medicale Can. 14 Apr 2009;180(8):814-20.
41. Yin P, Jiang CQ, Cheng KK, Lam TH, Lam KH, Miller MR, et al. Passive smoking exposure and risk of COPD among adults in China: the Guangzhou Biobank Cohort Study. Lancet Lond Engl. 1 Sep 2007;370(9589):751-7.
42. Campos MA, Alazemi S, Zhang G, Wanner A, Sandhaus RA. Effects of a disease management programme in individuals with alpha-1 antitrypsin deficiency. COPD. Feb 2009;6(1):31-40.
43. Hunninghake GM, Cho MH, Tesfaigzi Y, Soto-Quiros ME, Avila L, Lasky-Su J, et al. *MMP12,* Lung Function, and COPD in High-Risk Populations. N Engl J Med. 31 Dec 2009;361(27):2599-608.
44. Cho MH, Boutaoui N, Klanderman BJ, Sylvia JS, Ziniti JP, Hersh CP, et al. Variants in FAM13A are associated with chronic obstructive pulmonary disease. Nat Genet. March 2010;42(3):200-2.
45. Cho MH, McDonald M-LN, Zhou X, Mattheisen M, Castaldi PJ, Hersh CP, et al. Risk loci for chronic obstructive pulmonary disease: a genome-wide association study and metaanalysis. Lancet Respir Med. March 2014;2(3):214-25.
46. Hnizdo E, Sullivan PA, Bang KM, Wagner G. Association between chronic obstructive pulmonary disease and employment by industry and occupation in the US population: a study of data from the Third National Health and Nutrition Examination Survey. Am J Epidemiol. 15 Oct 2002;156(8):738-46.
47. American Thoracic Society Statement: Occupational Contribution to the Burden of Airway Disease. Am J Respir Crit Care Med. March 2003;167(5):787-97.
48. Gan WQ, FitzGerald JM, Carlsten C, Sadatsafavi M, Brauer M. Associations of ambient air pollution with chronic obstructive pulmonary disease hospitalization and mortality. Am J Respir Crit Care Med. 1 Apr 2013;187(7):721-7.
49. Paulin LM, Diette GB, Blanc PD, Putcha N, Eisner MD, Kanner RE, et al. Occupational Exposures Are Associated with Worse Morbidity in Patients with Chronic Obstructive Pulmonary Disease. Am J Respir Crit Care Med. March 2015;191(5):557-65.
50. Sunyer J, Spix C, Quénel P, Ponce-de-León A, Pönka A, Barumandzadeh T, et al. Urban air pollution and emergency admissions for asthma in four European cities: the APHEA

Project. Thorax. Sept 1997;52(9):760-5.
51. Atkinson RW, Anderson HR, Sunyer J, Ayres J, Baccini M, Vonk JM, et al. Acute effects of particulate air pollution on respiratory admissions: results from APHEA 2 project. Air Pollution and Health: a European Approach. Am J Respir Crit Care Med. 15 Nov 2001;164(10 Pt 1):1860-6.
52. Beran D, Zar HJ, Perrin C, Menezes AM, Burney P, Forum of International Respiratory Societies working group collaboration. Burden of asthma and chronic obstructive pulmonary disease and access to essential medicines in low-income and middle-income countries. Lancet Respir Med. Feb 2015;3(2):159-70.
53. Gershon AS, Warner L, Cascagnette P, Victor JC, To T. Lifetime risk of developing chronic obstructive pulmonary disease: a longitudinal population study. Lancet Lond Engl. 10 Sep 2011;378(9795):991-6.
54. Todisco T, de Benedictis FM, Iannacci L, Baglioni S, Eslami A, Todisco E, et al. Mild prematurity and respiratory functions. Eur J Pediatr. Jan 1993;152(1):55-8.
55. Lawlor DA. Association of birth weight with adult lung function: findings from the British Women's Heart and Health Study and a meta-analysis. Thorax. 1 Oct 2005;60(10):851-8.
56. Drummond MB, Kirk GD. HIV-associated obstructive lung diseases: insights and implications for the clinician. Lancet Respir Med. Jul 2014;2(7):583-92.
57. Byrne AL, Marais BJ, Mitnick CD, Lecca L, Marks GB. Tuberculosis and chronic respiratory disease: a systematic review. Int J Infect Dis IJID Off Publ Int Soc Infect Dis. March 2015;32:138-46.
58. Miravitlles M, Worth H, Soler Cataluña JJ, Price D, De Benedetto F, Roche N, et al. Observational study to characterise 24-hour COPD symptoms and their relationship with patient-reported outcomes: results from the ASSESS study. Respir Res. 21 Oct 2014;15:122.
59. Ofir D, Laveneziana P, Webb KA, Lam Y-M, O'Donnell DE. Mechanisms of dyspnea during cycle exercise in symptomatic patients with GOLD stage I chronic obstructive pulmonary disease. Am J Respir Crit Care Med. 2008 Mar 15;177(6):622-9.
60. Elbehairy AF, Ciavaglia CE, Webb KA, Guenette JA, Jensen D, Mourad SM, et al. Pulmonary Gas Exchange Abnormalities in Mild Chronic Obstructive Pulmonary Disease. Implications for Dyspnea and Exercise Intolerance. Am J Respir Crit Care Med. June 15, 2015;191(12):1384-94.
61. Barnes PJ, Celli BR. Systemic manifestations and comorbidities of COPD. Eur Respir J. May 2009;33(5):1165-85.
62. Maltais F, Leblanc P, Jobin J, Casaburi R. Peripheral muscle dysfunction in chronic obstructive pulmonary disease. Rev Mal Respir. Sept 2002;19(No 4):444-53.
63. O'Donnell DE, Banzett RB, Carrieri-Kohlman V, Casaburi R, Davenport PW, Gandevia SC, et al. Pathophysiology of dyspnea in chronic obstructive pulmonary disease: a roundtable. Proc Am Thorac Soc. May 2007;4(2):145-68.
64. Cho S-H, Lin H-C, Ghoshal AG, Bin Abdul Muttalif AR, Thanaviratananich S, Bagga S, et al. Respiratory disease in the Asia-Pacific region: Cough as a key symptom. Allergy Asthma Proc. Apr 2016;37(2):131-40.
65. Soler N, Esperatti M, Ewig S, Huerta A, Agustí C, Torres A. Sputum purulence-guided antibiotic use in hospitalised patients with exacerbations of COPD. Eur Respir J. Dec

2012;40(6):1344-53.
66. Brusse-Keizer MGJ, Grotenhuis AJ, Kerstjens H a. M, Telgen MC, van der Palen J, Hendrix MGR, et al. Relation of sputum colour to bacterial load in acute exacerbations of COPD. Respir Med. Apr 2009;103(4):601-6.
67. Stockley RA, O'Brien C, Pye A, Hill SL. Relationship of sputum colour to nature and outpatient management of acute exacerbations of COPD. Chest. June 2000;117(6):1638-45.
68. von Haehling S, Anker SD. Cachexia as a major underestimated and unmet medical need: facts and numbers. J Cachexia Sarcopenia Muscle. Sept 2010;1(1):1-5.
69. Schols AM, Soeters PB, Dingemans AM, Mostert R, Frantzen PJ, Wouters EF. Prevalence and characteristics of nutritional depletion in patients with stable COPD eligible for pulmonary rehabilitation. Am Rev Respir Dis. May 1993;147(5):1151-6.
70. Rutten EPA, Calverley PMA, Casaburi R, Agusti A, Bakke P, Celli B, et al. Changes in body composition in patients with chronic obstructive pulmonary disease: do they influence patient-related outcomes? Ann Nutr Metab. 2013;63(3):239-47.
71. Schols AMWJ, Broekhuizen R, Weling-Scheepers CA, Wouters EF. Body composition and mortality in chronic obstructive pulmonary disease. Am J Clin Nutr. Jul 2005;82(1):53-9.
72. Holleman DR, Simel DL. Does the Clinical Examination Predict Airflow Limitation? JAMA. 25 Jan 1995;273(4):313-9.
73. Kesten S, Chapman KR. Physician perceptions and management of COPD. Chest. July 1993;104(1):254-8.
74. Lamprecht B, McBurnie MA, Vollmer WM, Gudmundsson G, Welte T, Nizankowska-Mogilnicka E, et al. COPD in never smokers: results from the population-based burden of obstructive lung disease study. CHEST J. 2011;139(4):752-763.
75. Janson C, Marks G, Buist S, Gnatiuc L, Gislason T, McBurnie MA, et al. The impact of COPD on health status: findings from the BOLD study. Eur Respir J. Dec 2013;42(6):1472-83.
76. Al Ghobain M, Alhamad EH, Alorainy HS, Al Kassimi F, Lababidi H, Al-Hajjaj MS. The prevalence of chronic obstructive pulmonary disease in Riyadh, Saudi Arabia: a BOLD study. Int J Tuberc Lung Dis. 1 Oct 2015;19(10):1252-7.
77. Güder G, Brenner S, Angermann CE, Ertl G, Held M, Sachs AP, et al. GOLD or lower limit of normal definition? a comparison with expert-based diagnosis of chronic obstructive pulmonary disease in a prospective cohort-study. Respir Res. 2012;13(1):13.
78. Fishman A, Martinez F, Naunheim K, Piantadosi S, Wise R, Ries A, et al. A randomized trial comparing lung-volume-reduction surgery with medical therapy for severe emphysema. N Engl J Med. May 22, 2003;348(21):2059-73.
79. Klooster K, ten Hacken NHT, Hartman JE, Kerstjens HAM, van Rikxoort EM, Slebos DJ. Endobronchial Valves for Emphysema without Interlobar Collateral Ventilation. N Engl J Med. 10 Dec 2015;373(24):2325-35.
80. Amalakanti S, Pentakota MR. Pulse Oximetry Overestimates Oxygen Saturation in COPD. Respir Care. Apr 2016;61(4):423-7.
81. Kelly AM, McAlpine R, Kyle E. How accurate are pulse oximeters in patients with acute exacerbations of chronic obstructive airways disease? Respir Med. May 2001;95(5):336-40.
82. Cuvelier A. Alpha-1 antitrypsin deficiency. Oct 2007;24:7-17.

83. Bahloul N, Kallel N, Ketata W, Gargouri R, Moussa N, Kammoun S. Impact of COPD on patients' quality of life. Rev Mal Respir. 34:A150-1.
84. van den Boom G, Rutten-van Mölken MP, Tirimanna PR, van Schayck CP, Folgering H, van Weel C. Association between health-related quality of life and consultation for respiratory symptoms: results from the DIMCA programme. Eur Respir J. Jan 1998;11(1):67-72.
85. Seemungal TA, Donaldson GC, Paul EA, Bestall JC, Jeffries DJ, Wedzicha JA. Effect of exacerbation on quality of life in patients with chronic obstructive pulmonary disease. Am J Respir Crit Care Med. May 1998;157(5 Pt 1):1418-22.
86. Doll H, Miravitlles M. Health-related QOL in acute exacerbations of chronic bronchitis and chronic obstructive pulmonary disease: a review of the literature. PharmacoEconomics. 2005;23(4):345-63.
87. van der Molen T, Willemse BWM, Schokker S, ten Hacken NHT, Postma DS, Juniper EF. Development, validity and responsiveness of the Clinical COPD Questionnaire. Health Qual Life Outcomes. 28 Apr 2003;1:13.
88. Jones PW. Health status measurement in chronic obstructive pulmonary disease. Thorax. Nov 2001;56(11):880-7.
89. Jones PW, Quirk FH, Baveystock CM. The St George's Respiratory Questionnaire. Respir Med. Sept 1991;85 Suppl B:25-31; discussion 33-37.
90. Leplege A, Perneger T, Ecosse E, Pouchot J, Coste J. Le questionnaire MOS SF-36 : manuel de l'utilisateur et guide d'interprétation des scores. ISBN. 2001;155:118-5.
91. Jones PW, Harding G, Berry P, Wiklund I, Chen W-H, Kline Leidy N. Development and first validation of the COPD Assessment Test. Eur Respir J. Sept 2009;34(3):648-54.
92. Mahler DA, Mackowiak JI. Evaluation of the short-form 36-item questionnaire to measure health-related quality of life in patients with COPD. Chest. June 1995;107(6):1585-9.
93. Spencer S, Calverley PM, Sherwood Burge P, Jones PW. Health status deterioration in patients with chronic obstructive pulmonary disease. Am J Respir Crit Care Med. 2001;163(1):122-128.
94. Hajiro T, Nishimura K, Tsukino M, Ikeda A, Oga T, Izumi T. A comparison of the level of dyspnea vs disease severity in indicating the health-related quality of life of patients with COPD. Chest. Dec 1999;116(6):1632-7.
95. Barnes N, Calverley PMA, Kaplan A, Rabe KF. Chronic obstructive pulmonary disease and exacerbations: patient insights from the global Hidden Depths of COPD survey. BMC Pulm Med. 23 August 2013;13:54.
96. Watz H, Waschki B, Boehme C, Claussen M, Meyer T, Magnussen H. Extrapulmonary effects of chronic obstructive pulmonary disease on physical activity: a cross-sectional study. Am J Respir Crit Care Med. 1 Apr 2008;177(7):743-51.
97. Watz H, Waschki B, Kirsten A, Müller K-C, Kretschmar G, Meyer T, et al. The metabolic syndrome in patients with chronic bronchitis and COPD: frequency and associated consequences for systemic inflammation and physical inactivity. Chest. Oct 2009;136(4):1039-46.
98. Ford ES, Schulze MB, Pischon T, Bergmann MM, Joost H-G, Boeing H. Metabolic syndrome and risk of incident diabetes: findings from the European Prospective Investigation

into Cancer and Nutrition-Potsdam Study. Cardiovasc Diabetol. 12 Dec 2008;7:35.
99. Bolton CE, Ionescu AA, Shiels KM, Pettit RJ, Edwards PH, Stone MD, et al. Associated loss of fat-free mass and bone mineral density in chronic obstructive pulmonary disease. Am J Respir Crit Care Med. 15 Dec 2004;170(12):1286-93.
100.Sevenoaks MJ, Stockley RA. Chronic Obstructive Pulmonary Disease, inflammation and co-morbidity - a common inflammatory phenotype? Respir Res. 2006;7(1):70.
101.Similowski T, Agustí A, MacNee W, Schönhofer B. The potential impact of anaemia of chronic disease in COPD. Eur Respir J. Feb 2006;27(2):390-6.
102.Horwich TB, Fonarow GC, Hamilton MA, MacLellan WR, Borenstein J. Anemia is associated with worse symptoms, greater impairment in functional capacity and a significant increase in mortality in patients with advanced heart failure. J Am Coll Cardiol. June 5, 2002;39(11):1780-6.
103.Norwood RJ. A review of etiologies of depression in COPD. Int J Chron Obstruct Pulmon Dis. 2007;2(4):485-91.
104.Almagro P, Barreiro B, Ochoa de Echaguen A, Quintana S, Rodríguez Carballeira M, Heredia JL, et al. Risk factors for hospital readmission in patients with chronic obstructive pulmonary disease. Respir Int Rev Thorac Dis. 2006;73(3):311-7.
105.Xu W, Collet J-P, Shapiro S, Lin Y, Yang T, Platt RW, et al. Independent effect of depression and anxiety on chronic obstructive pulmonary disease exacerbations and hospitalizations. Am J Respir Crit Care Med. 2008 Nov 1;178(9):913-20.
106.Yohannes AM, Baldwin RC, Connolly MJ. Predictors of 1-year mortality in patients discharged from hospital following acute exacerbation of chronic obstructive pulmonary disease. Age Ageing. Sept 2005;34(5):491-6.
107.Ulubay G, Ulasli SS, Bozbas SS, Ozdemirel T, Karatas M. Effects of peripheral neuropathy on exercise capacity and quality of life in patients with chronic obstructive pulmonary diseases. Arch Med Sci AMS. May 9, 2012;8(2):296-302.
108.Voll-Aanerud M, Eagan TML, Wentzel-Larsen T, Gulsvik A, Bakke PS. Respiratory symptoms, COPD severity, and health related quality of life in a general population sample. Respir Med. March 2008;102(3):399-406.
109.Huiart L, Ernst P, Suissa S. Cardiovascular morbidity and mortality in COPD. Chest. Oct 2005;128((4)):2640-6.
110.Sin DD, Man SFP. Why are patients with chronic obstructive pulmonary disease at increased risk of cardiovascular diseases? The potential role of systemic inflammation in chronic obstructive pulmonary disease. Circulation. March 25, 2003;107(11):1514-9.
111.Hansell AL, Walk JA, Soriano JB. What do chronic obstructive pulmonary disease patients die from? A multiple cause coding analysis. Eur Respir J. Nov 2003;22(5):809-14.
112.Falk JA, Kadiev S, Criner GJ, Scharf SM, Minai OA, Diaz P. Cardiac disease in chronic obstructive pulmonary disease. Proc Am Thorac Soc. 1 May 2008;5(4):543-8.
113.Marquis K, Maltais F, Poirier P. [Cardiovascular manifestations in patients with COPD]. Rev Mal Respir. June 2008;25(6):663-73.
114.Fletcher C, Peto R. The natural history of chronic airflow obstruction. Br Med J. 1977;1(6077):1645-1648.
115.Tomczyk S, Bennett NM, Stoecker C, Gierke R, Moore MR, Whitney CG, et al. Use of 13valent pneumococcal conjugate vaccine and 23-valent pneumococcal polysaccharide

vaccine among adults aged >65 years: recommendations of the Advisory Committee on Immunization Practices (ACIP). MMWR Morb Mortal Wkly Rep. Sep 19, 2014;63(37):822-5.

116.Bonten MJM, Huijts SM, Bolkenbaas M, Webber C, Patterson S, Gault S, et al. Polysaccharide Conjugate Vaccine against Pneumococcal Pneumonia in Adults. N Engl J Med. March 19, 2015;372(12):1114-25.

117.Burge P, Calverley P, Jones P, Spencer S, Anderson J, Maslen T. Randomised, double blind, placebo controlled study of fluticasone propionate in patients with moderate to severe chronic obstructive pulmonary dise... BMJ. 13 May 2000;320(7245):1297-303.

118.Melani AS. Long-acting muscarinic antagonists. Expert Rev Clin Pharmacol. 2015;8(4):479-501.

119.Jones PW, Singh D, Bateman ED, Agusti A, Lamarca R, de Miquel G, et al. Efficacy and safety of twice-daily aclidinium bromide in COPD patients: the ATTAIN study. Eur Respir J. Oct 2012;40(4):830-6.

120.Karner C, Chong J, Poole P. Tiotropium versus placebo for chronic obstructive pulmonary disease. Cochrane Database Syst Rev. 11 Jul 2012;(7):CD009285.

121.Kesten S, Casaburi R, Kukafka D, Cooper CB. Improvement in self-reported exercise participation with the combination of tiotropium and rehabilitative exercise training in COPD patients. Int J Chron Obstruct Pulmon Dis. 2008;3(1):127-36.

122.Cazzola M, Molimard M. The scientific rationale for combining long-acting beta2-agonists and muscarinic antagonists in COPD. Pulm Pharmacol Ther. August 2010;23(4):257-67.

123.Wedzicha JA, Decramer M, Ficker JH, Niewoehner DE, Sandström T, Taylor AF, et al. Analysis of chronic obstructive pulmonary disease exacerbations with the dual bronchodilator QVA149 compared with glycopyrronium and tiotropium (SPARK): a randomised, double-blind, parallel-group study. Lancet Respir Med. May 2013;1(3):199-209.

124.Franssen FME, Wouters EFM, Vanfleteren LEGW. Indacaterol-Glycopyrronium for COPD. N Engl J Med. Sep 1, 2016;375(9):898-9.

125.Boardman C, Chachi L, Gavrila A, Keenan CR, Perry MM, Xia YC, et al. Mechanisms of glucocorticoid action and insensitivity in airways disease. Pulm Pharmacol Ther. dec 2014;29(2):129-43.

126.Yang IA, Clarke MS, Sim EHA, Fong KM. Inhaled corticosteroids for stable chronic obstructive pulmonary disease. Cochrane Database Syst Rev. 11 Jul 2012;(7):CD002991.

127.Vestbo J, Papi A, Corradi M, Blazhko V, Montagna I, Francisco C, et al. Single inhaler extrafine triple therapy versus long-acting muscarinic antagonist therapy for chronic obstructive pulmonary disease (TRINITY): a double-blind, parallel group, randomised controlled trial. Lancet Lond Engl. 13 May 2017;389(10082):1919-29.

128.Lipson DA, Barnacle H, Birk R, Brealey N, Locantore N, Lomas DA, et al. FULFIL Trial: Once-Daily Triple Therapy for Patients with Chronic Obstructive Pulmonary Disease. Am J Respir Crit Care Med. Aug 15, 2017;196(4):438-46.

129.Aubier M. Pharmacotherapy of respiratory muscles. Clin Chest Med. June 1988;9(2):311-24.

130.Moxham J. Aminophylline and the respiratory muscles: an alternative view. Clin Chest Med. June 1988;9(2):325-36.

131.ZuWallack RL, Mahler DA, Reilly D, Church N, Emmett A, Rickard K, et al. Salmeterol plus theophylline combination therapy in the treatment of COPD. Chest. June 2001;119(6):1661-70.

132.Zacarias EC, Castro AA, Cendon S. Effect of theophylline associated with short-acting or long-acting inhaled beta2-agonists in patients with stable chronic obstructive pulmonary disease: a systematic review. J Bras Pneumol. Apr 2007;33(2):152-60.

133.Rabe KF. Update on roflumilast, a phosphodiesterase 4 inhibitor for the treatment of chronic obstructive pulmonary disease. Br J Pharmacol. May 2011;163(1):53-67.

134.Calverley PMA, Rabe KF, Goehring U-M, Kristiansen S, Fabbri LM, Martinez FJ, et al. Roflumilast in symptomatic chronic obstructive pulmonary disease: two randomised clinical trials. Lancet Lond Engl. August 29, 2009;374(9691):685-94.

135.Fabbri LM, Calverley PMA, Izquierdo-Alonso JL, Bundschuh DS, Brose M, Martinez FJ, et al. Roflumilast in moderate-to-severe chronic obstructive pulmonary disease treated with longacting bronchodilators: two randomised clinical trials. Lancet Lond Engl. August 29, 2009;374(9691):695-703.

136.Murphy PB, Rehal S, Arbane G, Bourke S, Calverley PMA, Crook AM, et al. Effect of Home Noninvasive Ventilation With Oxygen Therapy vs Oxygen Therapy Alone on Hospital Readmission or Death After an Acute COPD Exacerbation: A Randomized Clinical Trial. JAMA. 06 2017;317(21):2177-86.

137.Han J, Dai L, Zhong N. Indacaterol on dyspnea in chronic obstructive pulmonary disease: a systematic review and meta-analysis of randomized placebo-controlled trials. BMC Pulm Med. 25 Apr 2013;13:26.

138.Cazzola M, Rogliani P, Ruggeri P, Segreti A, Proietto A, Picciolo S, et al. Chronic treatment with indacaterol and airway response to salbutamol in stable COPD. Respir Med. June 2013;107(6):848-53.

139.Leuppi JD, Schuetz P, Bingisser R, Bodmer M, Briel M, Drescher T, et al. Short-term vs conventional glucocorticoid therapy in acute exacerbations of chronic obstructive pulmonary disease: the REDUCE randomized clinical trial. JAMA. 5 June 2013;309(21):2223-31.

140.HAS recommendations. Therapeutic patient education. Definition, aims and organisation. 2007.

141.Bellamy D, Smith J. Role of primary care in early diagnosis and effective management of COPD: Role of primary care in COPD management. Int J Clin Pract. 10 Jul 2007;61(8):1380-9.

142.Darmon D, Roche N, Ghasarossian C, Stach B, Cittée J, Housset B. Detection of COPD in general practice: what perspective? Rev Mal Respir. Feb 2015;32(2):94-6.

143.Weltgesundheitsorganisation, publisher. Therapeutic patient education: continuing education programmes for health care providers in the field of prevention of chronic diseases; report of a WHO working group. Copenhagen; 1998. 77 p. (European health21 target 18, Developing human resources for health).

144.Lenferink A, Brusse-Keizer M, van der Valk PD, Frith PA, Zwerink M, Monninkhof EM, et al. Self-management interventions including action plans for exacerbations versus usual care in patients with chronic obstructive pulmonary disease. Cochrane Database Syst Rev. 4 Aug 2017;8:CD011682.

145.McGeoch GRB, Willsman KJ, Dowson CA, Town GI, Frampton CM, McCartin FJ, et al.

Self-management plans in the primary care of patients with chronic obstructive pulmonary disease. Respirol Carlton Vic. Sep 2006;11(5):611-8.

146.Rasekaba TM, Williams E, Hsu-Hage B. Can a chronic disease management pulmonary rehabilitation program for COPD reduce acute rural hospital utilization? Chron Respir Dis. 2009;6(3):157-63.

147.Leung J, Bhutani M, Leigh R, Pelletier D, Good C, Sin DD. Empowering family physicians to impart proper inhaler teaching to patients with chronic obstructive pulmonary disease and asthma. Can Respir J. Oct 2015;22(5):266-70.

148.Gagnayre R, Traynard PY. L'éducation du patient atteint de maladie chronique L'exemple du diabète. Actual Doss En Santé Publique. 2001;(36):48-49.

149.Atsou K, Chouaid C, Hejblum G. Simulation-Based Estimates of Effectiveness and Cost-Effectiveness of Smoking Cessation in Patients with Chronic Obstructive Pulmonary Disease. Su Z, editor. PLoS ONE. 14 Sep 2011;6(9):e24870.

150.Fournier C, Attali C. Éducation (thérapeutique) du patient en médecine générale. Médecine. 2012;8(3):123-128.

151.Miravitlles M, de la Roza C, Morera J, Montemayor T, Gobartt E, Martín A, et al. Chronic respiratory symptoms, spirometry and knowledge of COPD among general population. Respir Med. Nov 2006;100(11):1973-80.

152.Jébrak G, Vicaire M, Murez A. COPD: patients talk to carers. Survey by the Fédération française des associations et amicales de malades insuffisants ou handicapés respiratoires (FFAAIR). Rev Mal Respir. May 2015;32(5):500-12.

153.Emery CF, Schein RL, Hauck ER, MacIntyre NR. Psychological and cognitive outcomes of a randomized trial of exercise among patients with chronic obstructive pulmonary disease. Health Psychol Off J Div Health Psychol Am Psychol Assoc. May 1998;17(3):232-40.

154.Gibbons FX, Eggleston TJ, Benthin AC. Cognitive reactions to smoking relapse: the reciprocal relation between dissonance and self-esteem. J Pers Soc Psychol. Jan 1997;72(1):184-95.

155.Halpern MT. Effect of smoking characteristics on cognitive dissonance in current and former smokers. Addict Behav. Apr 1994;19(2):209-17.

156.Yawn BP, Wollan PC. Knowledge and attitudes of family physicians coming to COPD continuing medical education. Int J Chron Obstruct Pulmon Dis. 2008;3(2):311-7.

157.Walters N, Coleman T. Comparison of the smoking behaviour and attitudes of smokers who attribute respiratory symptoms to smoking with those who do not. Br J Gen Pr. 2002;52(475):132-134.

158.Jakoubovitch S, Bournot M-C, Cercier E, Tuffreau F. Les emplois du temps des médecins généralistes. Etudes Résultats. 2012;(797).

159.Foucaud J, Moquet MJ, Rostan F, Hamel E. État des lieux de la formation initiale en éducation thérapeutique du patient en France: résultats d'une analyse globale pour 10 professions de Santé. Evolutions. aVRIL 2008;12.

Appendix 1

Questionnaire "Therapeutic education of patients with COPD by general practitioners".

Questionnaire no. :

Profile of the doctor interviewed :

Age :

Sex: Male - Female

Type of practice: solo - group

Practice environment: urban - semi-rural - rural

Special exercise: no - yes (which one?)

Condition of the premises :

1. How would you define your role in relation to COPD patients?

□ Prevention □ Screening DSuivi- treatment □ Acute management

□ Education Advice Other - please specify

2. Do you provide therapeutic education for COPD patients?

□ Yes □ No

If YES

3. What do you do in practice?

3.1.Which speaker? □ You □ Other- Which one :

3.2.Is the patient accompanied? □ Yes No

3.3.Where? □ At the practice Other- Specify:

3.4.Are you in an advisory capacity? DOui□ No

3.5.Prescription? Yes □ No

3.6.How often do you monitor? □ Regular □ Irregular

How often (/quarter) :

4. Which organisation offering this service do you know?

□ None DEcole de l'Isthme/BPCO □ Other- Specify:

5. In your opinion, what are the aims and objectives of therapeutic education?

If NO

6. Why don't you do it?

GPs and ET :

7. Do you think this business should be expanded?

□ Don't know DOui □ No- Why :

If YES,

8. In what form?

8.1.Which speaker(s) :

□ General practitioner □ IDE specialising in therapeutic education

□ Respirologist DPsychologist □Kinesitherapist □ Other- Specify:
8.2.Where : □ At the practice DAl'hòpital Both □ Other- Specify:
8.3.How often: □ Regularly □ Not regularly
How often (/quarter)
8.4.What tools :
□ Evaluation questionnaire □ Follow-up booklet □ Visual aid □ Other - specify :

9. Which of the following key patient objectives should be achieved?
□ Awareness of the disease Knowledge about the disease
□ Their competence in terms of disease management
□ Other- Specify:
The COPD patient :
10. In your opinion, is there a demand from patients for this type of care?
? □ Yes No
If YES
11. What are their expectations?
□ Symptom relief Acute exacerbation management
□ Prevention of worsening and exacerbations □ Self-management Other - specify:
If NO
12. Why is this?
Conclusion:
13. What are your expectations in terms of therapeutic education?

Appendix 2

Bristol COPD Knowledge Questionnaire (BCKQ)

R White et al (2008)

			True	False	Don't know
1.	**In COPD:**				
	a.	In COPD the word "chronic" means it is severe	O	X	O
	b.	COPD can only be confirmed by breathing tests	X	O	O
	c.	In COPD there is usually gradual worsening over time	X	O	O
	d.	In COPD oxygen levels in the blood are always low	O	X	O
	e.	COPD is unusual in people less than 40 years old	X	O	O
2.	**COPD :**				
	a.	More than 80% of COPD cases are caused by cigarette smoking	X	O	O
	b.	COPD can be caused by occupational dust exposure	X	O	O
	c.	Longstanding asthma can develop into COPD	X	O	O
	d.	COPD is commonly an inherited disease	O	X	O
	e.	Women are less vulnerable to the effects of cigarette smokingthan men	O	X	O
3.	**The following symptoms are common in COPD :**				
	a.	Swelling of ankles	O	X	O
	b.	Tiredness	X	O	O
	c.	Wheezing	X	O	O
	d.	Crushing chest pain	O	X	O
	e.	Rapid weight loss	O	X	O
4.	**Breathlessness in COPD :**				
	a.	Severe breathlessness prevents travel by air	O	X	O
	b.	Breathlessness can be worsened by eating large meals	X	O	O
	c.	Breathlessness means that your oxygen levels are low	O	X	O
	d.	Breathlessness is a normal response to exercise	X	O	O
	e.	Breathlessness is primarily caused by a narrowing of thebronchial tubes	X	O	O
5.	**Phlegm (sputum) :**				
	a.	Coughing phlegm is a common symptom in COPD	X	O	O
	b.	Clearing phlegm is more difficult if you get dehydrated	X	O	O
	c.	Bronchodilatator inhalers can help clear phlegm	X	O	O
	d.	Phlegm causes harm if swallowed	O	X	O
	e.	Clearing phlegm can be assisted by breathing exercises	X	O	O
6.	**Chest infections / Exacerbations :**				
	a.	Chest infections often cause coughing of blood	O	X	O
	b.	With chest infections phlegm usually becomes coloured (yellowor green)	X	O	O
	c.	Exacerbations (episodes of worsening) can occur in the absence of a chest infection	X	O	O
	d.	Chest infections are always associated with ahigh temperature	O	X	O
	e.	Steroids tablets should be taken whenever there isan exacerbation	O	X	O
7.	**Exercise in COPD :**				
	a.	Walking is better exercise than breathing exercises toimprove fitness	X	O	O
	b.	Exercise should be avoided as it strains the lungs	O	X	O
	c.	Exercise can help maintain your bone density	X	O	O
	d.	Exercise helps relieve depression	X	O	O
	e.	Exercise should be stopped if it makes you breathless	O	X	O
8.	**Smoking :**				
	a.	Stopping smoking will reduce the risk of heart disease	X	O	O
	b.	Stopping smoking will slow down further lung damage	X	O	O
	c.	Stopping smoking is pointless as the damage is done	O	X	O
	d.	Stopping smoking usually results in improved lung function	O	X	O
	e.	Nicotine replacement therapy is only available on prescription	O	X	O
9.	**Vaccination :**				
	a.	A flu jab is recommended every year	X	O	O
	b.	You can get flu from having a flu jab	O	X	O
	c.	You can only have a flu jab if you are 65 or over	O	X	O
	d.	A pneumonia jab protects against all forms of pneumonia	O	X	O
	e.	You can have a pneumonia jab and a flu jab on the same day	X	O	O
10.	**Inhaled Bronchodilators :**				
	a.	All bronchodilators act quickly (within 10 minutes)	O	X	O
	b.	Both short and long acting bronchodilators can be taken on the Saturday	X	O	O
	c.	Spacers (e.g. Nebuhaler, Aerochamber) should be dried with a towel after washing	O	X	O

d.	Using a spacer device will increase the amount of drug deposited in thelungs	X	O	O
e.	Tremor may be a side effect of bronchodilators	X	O	O
11. Antibiotic treatment in COPD :				
a.	To be effective, the course should last at least 10 days	O	X	O
b.	Excessive use of antibiotics can cause resistant bacteria (germs)	X	O	O
c.	Antibiotics will clear all chest infections	O	X	O
d.	Antibiotics treatment is necessary for an exacerbation (worsening) however mild	O	X	O
e.	You should seek advice if antibiotics cause severe diarrhea	X	O	O
12. Steroids tablets given for COPD (e.g. prednisolone)				
a.	Steroid tablets help strengthen muscles	O	X	O
b.	Steroid tablets should be avoided if there is a chest infections	O	X	O
c.	The risk of long-term side effects due to steroids is less with short courses than with continuoustreatment	X	O	O
d.	Indigestion is a common side effect from using steroid tablets	X	O	O
e.	Steroid tablets can increase your appetite	X	O	O
13. Inhaled Steroids (brown, red or orange)				
a.	Inhaled steroids should be stopped if you are given steroid tablets	O	X	O
b.	Steroid inhalers can be used for rapid relief of breathlessness	O	X	O
c.	Spacer devices reduce the risk of getting thrushed in themouth	X	O	O
d.	Steroid inhaler should be taken before your bronchodilator	O	X	O
e.	Inhaled steroids improve lung function in COPD	O	X	O

Appendix 3

Fletcher curve illustrating Karret's interest in tobacco

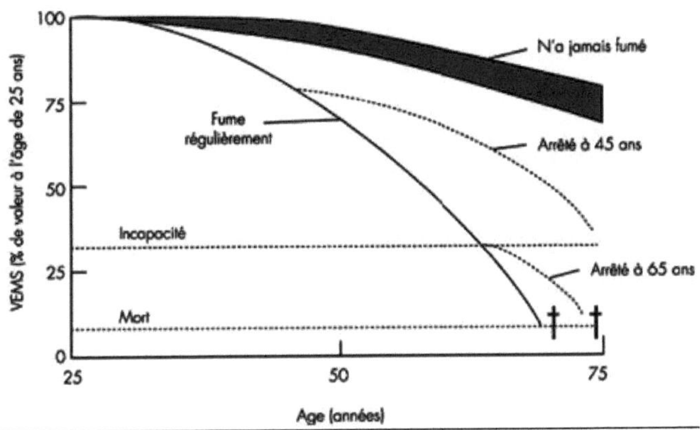

Age (years)

Age-related decline in FEV1

The grey area represents the physiological decline (noreceptive smoker or smoker unreceptive to the harmful effects of cigarettes), while the solid line represents the occult decline observed in the receptive smoker. The dotted line represents the decline, from age 45 onwards, in an ex-smoker who stopped smoking at the age of 45.

SUMMARY

INTRODUCTION

Chronic obstructive pulmonary disease represents a major challenge in terms of patient care, healthcare costs and quality of life. Like any chronic disease, it requires patients to adhere to the necessary treatment. However, this is not the case with chronic patients, who often do not adhere well to their treatments or to the advice given by their carers. Therapeutic patient education is the answer to this problem. It is a process that will enable patients to participate in improving their quality of life, while acquiring skills in adaptation and self-management. GPs, who are the primary care providers, are primarily responsible for delegating this therapeutic education to patients, willingly passing on their skills to them, which plays a crucial role in their perceptions of the disease, with a major impact on therapeutic management and the level of control of the disease.

AIMS OF THE STUDY

Given that the practice of therapeutic education with patients by GPs has not been evaluated, the aims of this study are to assess GPs' views on therapeutic education and to evaluate their theoretical knowledge and level of involvement in the overall management of chronic lung disease.

MATERIALS AND METHODS

This is a descriptive cross-sectional study which was carried out among general practitioners in the Sfax region over a period of 4 months. A first questionnaire was designed around three axes: disease management in general practice, therapeutic education in COPD and patient demand for the education process. A second questionnaire, the Bristol COPD knowledge questionnaire, was administered to doctors to assess their knowledge of chronic obstructive pulmonary disease.

RESULTS

The rate of correct responses to the questionnaire assessing doctors' knowledge was 72%.

As regards the functional signs of the disease, cough, dyspnoea and sputum are the most frequent symptoms according to our doctors.

To make a positive diagnosis of COPD, half the doctors used respiratory tests, while the other half relied on purely clinical criteria. Inadequate diagnosis of the disease is compounded by a lack of knowledge about COPD and its symptoms among the general population (60% of doctors thought that patients had only a very limited knowledge of the disease).

When it comes to COPD management, stopping smoking is the main therapeutic measure according to all respondents. The flu vaccine is known to be indicated annually, but influenza can occur (according to 66% of respondents). It was also noted that antibiotics and oral corticoids are still over-prescribed, irrespective of the severity of exacerbations and for periods exceeding international recommendations.

With regard to therapeutic education, two thirds of our doctors stated that they practised this approach mainly in their practices (94%) and during consultations (83%). This leads us to conclude that it was an implicit practice. In fact, the WHO recommends a structural programme representing a reference framework for implementing a personalised programme for each patient.

General practitioners and respirologists are the main players in therapeutic education, according to our doctors. Patients need education, but not all of them seek it (according to 45% of doctors).

All doctors are convinced of the need to promote the educational process in primary care. However, 33% of our respondents cited a number of barriers to this practice. Refusal to stop smoking by uncooperative patients was cited as the main obstacle. The lack of time and training for professionals and the absence of a coordinated network facilitating the integration of GPs into multidisciplinary care were also cited. GPs therefore need to be made aware of and trained in the issues and practice of education, and need to be better able to convince patients of the value of the educational approach.

CONCLUSION

Despite the progress made in the field of chronic diseases, chronic obstructive pulmonary disease is still a little-known disease and the poor relation of therapeutic education. The role of education should be better defined and clearly provided on a multidisciplinary basis, involving the GP for the benefit of the patient. We still need to set objectives that are tailored to the needs of doctors and patients...

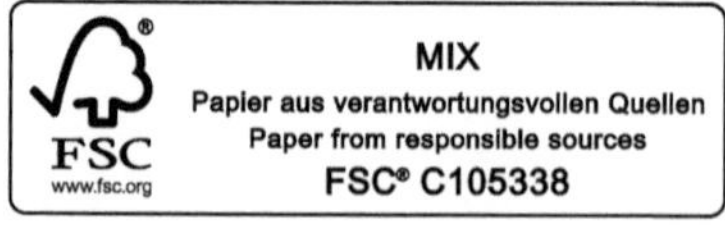

Printed by Books on Demand GmbH, Norderstedt / Germany